全国高等医学院校配套实验教材

BASIC MEDICAL CHEMISTRY EXPERIMENT

医用基础化学实验

（英文版）

Editors　Sun Lian　Chang Junmin
主　编　孙　莲　常军民

Associate editor　Hailiqian Taoerdahon
副主编　海力茜·陶尔大洪

Join editors　Ma Xiaoli　Li Gairu　Ainiwaer　Wang Yan
　　　　　　Zhang Xuan　Meng Lei　Yao Jun
编　委　马晓丽　李改茹　艾尼娃尔　王　岩
　　　　张　煊　孟　磊　姚　军

科学出版社
北京

内 容 简 介

本书为英文版医用基础化学实验教材,是医学院校本科生医用化学方法的基础教学,为培养学生的科学思维方法而编写的。全书内容包括:实验的一般规则、实验报告的格式及21个基础化学实验。特点是:英文教学,适用性强,具有科学性、创新性。

本书可适用于全国高等医学院校本科生用。

图书在版编目(CIP)数据

医用基础化学实验:英文版 = BASIC MEDICAL CHEMISTRY EXPERIMENT/孙莲,常军民主编. —北京:科学出版社,2007
全国高等医学院校配套实验教材
ISBN 9787-03-017924-1

Ⅰ. 医… Ⅱ. ①孙…②常… Ⅲ. 医用化学－化学实验－医学院校－教材－英文 Ⅳ. R313-33

中国版本图书馆 CIP 数据核字(2006)第 100871 号

责任编辑:郭海燕　夏　宇／责任校对:桂伟利
责任印制:徐晓晨／封面设计:黄　超

版权所有,违者必究。未经本社许可,数字图书馆不得使用

科 学 出 版 社 出版
北京东黄城根北街16号
邮政编码:100717
http://www.sciencep.com

北京厚诚则铭印刷科技有限公司 印刷
科学出版社发行　各地新华书店经销

*

2007年1月第 一 版　开本:B5(720×1000)
2016年8月第二次印刷　印张:6 1/2
字数:123 000

定价:29.80元
(如有印装质量问题,我社负责调换)

PREFACE

Experiment teaching is one of the most fundamental teaching to clinical medicine specialized students, playing an important role in training scientific thoughts and methods, creative consciousness and ability of the students as well as in promoting quality-oriented education in all-round way.

Based on the experience of medical basic chemistry experiment teaching for many years, by using for reference the experiments of inorganic chemistry and analytical chemistry in other colleges and universities, we have finished this textbook. The experiments in this textbook have the individuality, systematicness and scientificalness and emphasis the connecting with other experimental courses, which helps the foreign students to grasp basic techniques of operation within the class hours of experimental teaching prescribed by teaching syllabus and to improve their experimental ability and finally to cultivate a scientific approach of precision, practicality and creation.

21 experiments have been compiled, including 15 validate experiments, 5 comprehensive experiments and 1 designing experiment in this textbook. Validate experiments is on the training of basic experiments to intensify students' basic experiment skills and comprehensive experiment can train students' abilities in analyzing and solving complicated problem, designing experiment can improve students sense and ability of blazing new trails. Besides, after each experiment, we have compiled the preview; operation instructions, and points for attention, questions.

During compiling this textbook, we have tried our best to select suitable materials, however, there are still something improper or even erroneous due to our academic limitations. We would be most appreciative if anyone could give us good suggestions on improving this experimental textbook.

Editor
July 7 2006

CONTENTS

PREFACE
EXPERIMENTAL GENERAL RULE ············· (1)
EXPERIMENT REPORT FORMAT ············· (3)
EXPERIMENT ONE ············· (4)
   Weighing Exercise ············· (4)
EXPERIMENT TWO ············· (6)
   Acid-base Titration ············· (6)
EXPERIMENT THREE ············· (11)
   The Preparation and Standardization of 0.1mol/L Hydrochloride Acid Solution
   ············· (11)
EXPERIMENT FOUR ············· (14)
   The Preparation and Standardization of Sodium Hydroxide Solution ············· (14)
EXPERIMENT FIVE ············· (17)
   The Usage of Depression of Freezing Point to Determine the Molecular Weight
   of Glucose ············· (17)
EXPERIMENT SIX ············· (21)
   Determining the Ionization Constant of a Weak Acid ············· (21)
EXPERIMENT SEVEN ············· (25)
   Buffer Solution ············· (25)
EXPERIMENT EIGHT ············· (29)
   pH Measurement of Liquid Drug Preparation with pH Meter ············· (29)
EXPERIMENT NINE ············· (33)
   Precipitation Equilibrium ············· (33)
EXPERIMENT TEN ············· (38)
   Redox Reaction ············· (38)
EXPERIMENT ELEVEN ············· (43)
   Determination of Solubility Product of AgAc ············· (43)
EXPERIMENT TWELVE ············· (47)
   Determining the Coordination Number of $[Ag(NH_3)_n]^+$ ············· (47)

EXPERIMENT THIRTEEN .... (51)
　Coordination Compounds .... (51)
EXPERIMENT FOURTEEN .... (57)
　The Properties of Halogen .... (57)
EXPERIMENT FIFTEEN .... (62)
　Preparation of Medicinal Sodium Chloride and Examination of Impurities
　　Limitation .... (62)
EXPERIMENT SIXTEEN .... (69)
　Preparation of Ferrous Ammonium Sulfate Hexahydrate (FAS) .... (69)
EXPERIMENT SEVENTEEN .... (72)
　Preparation and Content Assay of Zinc Gluconate .... (72)
EXPERIMENT EIGHTEEN .... (75)
　Synthesis of Copper Sulfate Pentahydrate .... (75)
EXPERIMENT NINETEEN .... (78)
　Preparation of SnI_4 .... (78)
EXPERIMENT TWENTY .... (81)
　Separation and Identification of Methionine and Glycine by Paper Chromatography
　　............ (81)
EXPERIMENT TWENTY ONE .... (85)
　Synthesis of Potassium Permanganate .... (85)

EXERCISE .... (87)
APPENDIX .... (95)
　Table 1　List of Atomic Weight .... (95)
　Table 2　The Concentration of Acid and Base Used Frequently in Laboratory
　　............ (98)

EXPERIMENTAL GENERAL RULE

Laboratory rule

(1) To prepare a lesson earnestly before the experiment. To indicate clearly about the goal and request of the experiment. To clarify the related basic principle, sequence of the operation, and about safety in the experiment.

(2) To put on the working clothes before entering the laboratory. To maintain calm in the experimental process. Achieves the operation earnestly, observation carefully, positive ponder. Records the experimental phenomenon and the empirical data truthfully.

(3) Take care on state property. Uses the instrumentation and equipment carefully. Saves the drugs electricity and the water.

(4) In the laboratory bench instrument should neatly place at the suitable and position, and maintain the floor neat. Do not have the scrap paper, match sticks, damage glassware and so on to throw into the water trough in order to avoid stops up.

(5) When uses the precise instrument, it must strictly carry on the operation according to the working instruction. If the instrument has been destroyed, it should stop to use and report immediately to instruct teacher, promptly fixes the breakdown.

(6) After experiment, clean the used instrument neatly and return test apparatus in the cabinet. If it is damaged, promptly registered. And inspected by the teacher and registered on the primitive minute book, then leave the laboratory.

(7) After every test the student, being on duty for the day in turn is responsible for cleaning up the laboratory, inspecting the switch of water and electricity, and fastening the window. To maintain the laboratory neatness and its insecurity.

(8) After completing the experiment, the data should process earnestly and write the test report according to the primary record and related theoretical knowledge. Let the teacher to inspect on time.

The laboratory safety regulation

In chemistry experiment, some in flammable, explosive, violent, corrosive chemicals are contacted frequently. Some chemical reactions also have the risk. It uses frequently the water, electricity and many kinds of heating up the lamps and lanterns (such as alcohol lamp, gas lamp and so on). Therefore, when carries on chemistry experiment, the security problem must fully be taken in mind. Before experiment, understanding fully related security matters and take gread care to it. In the experimental process, observes the working instruction strictly in order to avoid the accident occurs.

(1) Every experiment of producing irritant, odor, violent gas should be carried on in the ventilation chamber(or ventilating place).

(2) The concentrate acids and alkali possess strong corrosiveness, these must be need carefully, be sure not to splash on clothes, on the skin and the eye. On diluting strong sulfuric acid, the acid should pour in slowly into the water with stirring , but water cannot pour into in the strong sulfuric acid.

(3) The virulent drugs (for example lead salt, arsenic compound, specially fluoride) cannot be entered into the mouth or the contact wound. These cannot be casually pour into the sewer and should pour into the vessel according to the teacher as requested.

(4) On heating up the test tube, never face any orifice of the test tube, also cannot overlook the liquid on heating to guard against the liquid to splash or offend somebody.

(5) It is not allow to handle solid drugs with the hand directly. When smells the gas, the nose cannot treat the bottle mouth or the orifice directly, but apply gently few gas to nostril carefully.

(6) Uses the alcohol lamp along with the spot. Strictly prohibits lighting other lamps with the burning alcohol lamp, in order to avoid the ethylalcohol flows out and catches fire.

(7) Uses the flammable and explosive drugs, strictly observes the working instruction, be far away the open fire.

(8) Does not allow to mix each kind of chemicals arbitrarily, in order to avoid possibly accident.

(9) The water, electricity, coal gas should be close immediately after use.

(10) In the laboratory, smoking and the diet should be strictly prohibits. After the experiment ended, cleans both hands and then leaves the laboratory.

Li Gairu

EXPERIMENT REPORT FORMAT

Experiment objective: _____　　　**Score:** _____

Profession, class: _____　　　**Name:** _____

Experiment date: _____ year _____ month _____ day

1. Experiment objective

2. Experiment principle

3. Experiment procedure

4. Experiment data recorded and the result expressed

5. Discuss

6. Questions

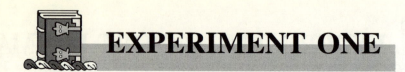

EXPERIMENT ONE

Weighing Exercise

Objectives

1. Exercise the correct weighing method: direct weighing, weighing by difference, weighing substance of fixed weight.

2. Learn to use analytical balance correctly.

Principle

The analytical balance is a first-class leve apparats to compare two masses. The principle of operation is based on the fact that at balance $M_1 L_1 = M_2 L_2$ (M_1 represents the unknown mass, M_2 represents a known mass, L_1 and L_2 represent arm length). As the two arms are constructed to be of the same length, therefore, at balance $M_1 = M_2$. A pointer is placed on the beam of the balance as an indicator when a state of balance is achieved. Before the operator adjusts the value of M_2 the balance should be unloaded until the pointer returns to its original position on the scale.

Equipment

Balance, a weighing bottle, a beaker (50mL or 100mL) or a conical flask (250mL).

Chemicals

NaCl.

Procedures

1. Direct weighing: place the object on the balance, and weigh it directly.

2. Weighing by difference: the sample in the weighing bottle is weighed and then a portion is removed (e. g. , by tapping) and quantitatively transferred to a vessel appropriate for dissolving the sample. The weighing bottle and the sample are then reweighed and the weight of sample is obtained from the difference. The weight of the next sample can be obtained by repeating the process.

3. Weighing an object of fixed weight: weigh the weighing paper (or weighing bottle, small beaker and so on) alone on the balance, then add sample with a clean spatula. Weigh the sample plus weighing paper. Subtract the weight of weighing paper to obtain the weight of the sample. This method is only valid for samples that do not absorb water from the air on standing.

Notes

1. Never place chemicals directly on the balance, but weigh them in a vessel (weighing bottle, weighing dish) or on filter paper. Always brash spilled chemicals off immediately with a soft brush.

2. Always close the balance case door before weighing. Air currents will cause the balance unsteady.

3. Weigh at room temperature, avoid air convection currents.

Questions

1. How to use significant figures in a weighing calculation?
2. How to weigh an object accurately and quickly?
3. In weighing by difference, do the zero point need to be set? Why?
4. Does the weight the weighing bottle lost exactly equal to the weight the beaker increased? Where does the difference come from?

Ainiwaer

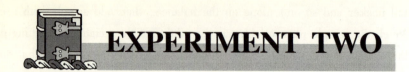

EXPERIMENT TWO

Acid-base Titration

Objectives

1. Practice the operation of titration.
2. Determine the concentration of sodium hydroxide solution and hydrochloric acid solution (mol/L).

Principle

The concentration of an acid or a base can be determined with the acid-base neutralization reaction. The most obvious application of neutralization method is to determine the amount of a base by titrating a measured amount of an acid. With the volume of the base added V_b and the original volume of the acid V_a and the concentration of acid C_a already known, we can calculate the concentration of base C_b.

$$C_a V_a = C_b V_b$$

Whereas, C_a can be calculated from V_a, V_b and C_b.

The equivalent point of the titration can be located by the color change of the acid-base indicator.

In this experiment, titrate the oxalic acid of exactly known concentration with NaOH solution, the concentration of NaOH can be obtained, then titrate the chloric acid with that NaOH solution, so the concentration of chloric acid can be obtained.

Equipment

Burette, pipette.

Chemicals

NaOH solution, HCl solution, oxalic acid standard solution, phenolphthaleins

Procedures

Standardizing the concentration of NaOH solution

Clean up the basic burette rinsed with distilled water and with NaOH solution for three times. Keep the burette level and carefully rotate it then let drop the solution out from the tip of the burette so that interior surface are wetted. After that, fill NaOH solution into it, drive away the air bubble in the rubber tube and its tip, then adjust the place of the liquid level to "0.00".

Add 20.00mL oxalic acid standard solution with transfer pipette to Erlenmeyer flask, then add 2—3 drops of phenolphthalein indicator, shaking constantly.

Extrude the glass ball in rubber tube to make the liquid dropping to Erlenmeyer flask. The dropping velocity can be quick at the beginning, but afterwards the operation should be controlled drop by drop and avoiding a current of liquid. When the base solution drops into the Erlenmeyer flask, part of the solution appears pink, but the color will disappear quickly while shaking the Erlenmeyer flask. pink color disappears slowly near the end-point. In this period the base solution should be added a drop at a time and allow a half drop of liquid hanging on the tip. It should not fall directly only make it touch the inner wall of the Erlenmeyer flask and then shake. If the pink color doesn't disappear in about half a minute, it means that the end-point is located. Wait a moment, then record the place of the liquid level left in the burette.

Titrate the oxalic acid standard solution with NaOH solution twice using the above method. The difference between the base volume added in every titration should be no more than 0.10mL.

You must pay attention to the following points:

(1) There should not be some droplet left out side the tip of burette and also there should not be some air bubbles left inside the tip when the titration is over.

(2) The color of the solution after the location of the end-point will disappear because of the effect of CO_2 in the open air. That doesn't mean the acid-base reaction is not complete.

(3) During the titration, the base may splash down the upper part of the wall of the Erlenmeyer flask and the last half drop is touched by the wall, so in the immediate vicinity of the end-point it is appropriate to rinse down before completing the titration.

Determining the concentration of HCl solution

Clean up the acidic burette rinsed with the distilled water and with HCl solution for three times. Then fill in the HCl solution and adjust the place of liquid level to "0.00"mL.

Add 20.00mL HCl solution to the Erlenmeyer flask from the acidic burette, then add 2—3 drops of phenolphthalein. Titrate it with NaOH solution according to the above operation. If an excess amount of NaOH is added, you can add HCl solution from the acidic burette until the red color disappears. Then titrate again. Record the volume of

HCl solution and NaOH solution added at the end-point.

Data result

1. Standardizing the concentration of NaOH solution (Table 1):

Table 1 Data result

experiment number	1	2	3
volume of NaOH/mL			
volume of oxalic acid/mL			
concentration of oxalic acid/(mol·L^{-1})			
concentration of NaOH/(mol·L^{-1})			
the average concentration of NaOH/(mol·L^{-1})			

2. Determining the concentration of HCl solution (Table 2):

Table 2 The concentration of HCl solution

experiment number	1	2	3
volume of NaOH/mL			
volume of HCl/mL			
concentration of HCl/(mol·L^{-1})			
the average concentration of HCl/(mol·L^{-1})			

Instructions

Requirements

(1) Go over the theory of acid-base neutralization reaction.

(2) Pay much attention to prepare how to wash the transfer pipette and how to operate with burette in "The basic operations in experimental inorganic chemistry".

(3) How to wash transfer pipette? Why should we clean it up with the solution filled in? Should we clean up the burette and erlenmeyer flask in the same way?

(4) Why should we drive away the air bubbles in the tip of the burette before filled in the liquid? If not, what's the result on reading the volume of the liquid?

(5) If some droplet is left outside the tip of burette after the titration, and some drops are splashed down on the wall of Erlenmeyer flask but not being rinsed with the distilled water, what's the effect on the result?

Operation

(1) Learn how to use the burette and the transfer pipette.

(2) Grasp the operation of acid-base titration.

Notes

(1) Smear some Vaseline on the two sides of the stopcock of the acidic burette and then insert the stopcock into the barred and rotate it vigorously. The burette should be liquid-tight. Take care not to smear the whole stopcock, otherwise the hole will be jammed.

(2) Steep the burette and the transfer pipette in hot chromic acid solution for about 10 minutes, then the chromic acid should be poured back to the original bottle. Because chromic acid is poisonous, so do not pour it to the sewer.

(3) Wash the burette and transfer pipette with tap water and distilled water, then clean up them with the solution that will be filled in.

(4) Place a forefinger of your right hand over the upper end of the pipette, then carefully fill the pipette somewhat past the graduation mark employing a suction bulb.

(5) Allow the liquid in the transfer pipette to flow out, it's better to leave the tip of transfer pipette to the inner wall of the Erlenmeyer flask for 30s, then take it away.

(6) Fill the standard solution into the burette to the place above the zero mark, then lower the level of the solution to "0.00" mL, after driving away the air bubbles in the rubber tube and the glass tip.

(7) The dropping velocity may be controlled a little quicker at the beginning of the titration. At this moment the pink color of the indicator will disappear immediately; near the end-point; pink color disappears slowly, It must titrate a drop at a time until pink color doesn't disappear in half minute. It means the end-point is located.

(8) No drop should be left outside the tip after the titration is over. The Erlenmeyer flask may be tipped with distilled water and rotated it so that the bulk of the liquid picks up any droplets adhering to the wall.

(9) Some droplets may be splashed down the wall of the Erlenmeyer flask during the titration, a little amount of distilled water from the washing bottle should be pressed to rinse the inner wall while approaching the end-point.

Report format

(1) Objectives.

(2) Principle.

(3) Record data and result dealing with:

(a) The standardization of the concentration of NaOH solution (Refer to the content and list with table shown in one or same page).

(b) The determination of the concentration of HCl solution (Refer to the content and list with table shown in one or same page).

Questions

(1) When titrating an acid with a base, does the color of the solution disappear again after the end-point is located if the indicator is phenolphthalein?

(2) The reason for error in this experiment.

Ainiwaer

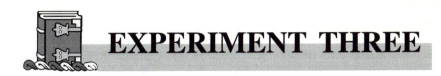
EXPERIMENT THREE

The Preparation and Standardization of 0.1mol/L Hydrochloride Acid Solution

Objectives

1. Master the principle and method of using sodium carbonate (Na_2CO_3) as the primary standard substance to standardize hydrochloride acid solution.

2. Properly judge tile ending point of Methy₁ red-bromocresol green as mixed indicator.

Principle

Hydrochloride acid is easy to volatize and the standardized solution can not be prepared directly. So solution of the approximate concentration should be made first, and then standardize it with primary standard substance.

The primary standard substance for standardize acid solution is anhydrous sodium carbonate (Na_2CO_3), or borate etc. In this copy anhydrous sodium carbonate is used as primacy standard substance and methyl red-bromocresol green mixed indicator as the indicator. At the ending point, the color changes from green to purple. The reaction is in the following equation:

$$2HCl + Na_2CO_3 = 2NaCl + H_2CO_3$$

According to the mass of the primary standard substance and the volume of hydrochloride acid consumed, the concentration of hydrochloride acid can be calculated from the following below equation:

$$C_{HCl} = \frac{2w_{Na_2CO_3}(g)}{V_{HCl} \cdot \frac{M_{Na_2CO_3}}{1000}}$$

$$M_{Na_2CO_3} = 105.99 \ (g/mol)$$

Equipment

Drop-burette (25mL), conical flask (250mL), volumetric cylinder (100mL, 10mL).

Chemicals

Standardized sodium carbonate reagent; hydrochloric acid: the concentration is about 36%—38%, relative density is 1.18; methy₁ red-bromocresol green mixed indicator; 3 portions of 0.1% bromcresol green and 1 portion of 0.2% methyl red is ethanol.

Procedure

Preparation of 0.1mol/L hydrochloric acid (HCl) solution

Transfer 9mL HCl to a flask with a stopper, dilute it with distilled water to 1 000mL and mix well.

Standardization of 0.1mol/L hydrochloric acid (HCl) solution

Weigh accurately about 0.12g of anhydrous Sodium carbonate (Na_2CO_3) which has previously been dried to constant weight at 270—290℃ in a conical flask. Dissolve it with 50mL distilled water and add 10 drops of methy₁ red-bromocresed green IS. Titrate it with 0.1mol/L HCl solution till the color change from green to violet red. Boil it for 2 minutes, then cool it to room temperature (or shaking by swirling for 2 minutes), Then titrate it from green to purple, that's the end-point.

Notes

1. Sodium Carbonate (Na_2CO_3) must be measured rapidly because it's easy to absorb water.

2. pH does not change greatly when it is close to the ending point and the ending point isn't perspicacity because it forms H_2CO_3-$NaHCO_3$ buffer solution. So the solution is boiled for 2 minutes then cool (or shaking by swirling it for 2minutes).

3. Be careful not to spill on boiling or shaking.

4. The color of the ending point changes from green→caesious→purple. When it is close to the ending point, shaking by swirling it for 2 minutes, the color of the solution changes back to green, go on titrating it slowly to purple. That's the ending point.

5. Use acid buret correctly, e.g., coating the piston with Vaseline, pushing away the bubble. The basic operation like how to control the half-drop or one-drop titration.

Questions

1. How to prepare 1 000mL HCl solution (0.1mol/L)?
2. Should all the conical flasks used for the experiment be free from water? Should

the distilled water used be accurately measured?

3. Why the solution has to be boiled when close to the ending point on using Na_2CO_3 to standardize HCl solution? And why has to cool it before titrating to the ending point?

4. How to calculate the quantity of the primary standard substance. When using Na_2CO_3 to standardize (0.1 mol/L) HCl solution?

Ainiwaer

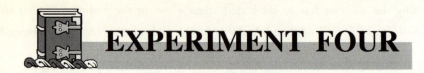

EXPERIMENT FOUR

The Preparation and Standardization of Sodium Hydroxide Solution

Objectives

1. Master the titration with an alkali type burette and the determination of the end point of a titration.

2. Learn how to prepare and standardization of solutions with primary standard substance.

Principle

Sodium hydroxide absorbs water and carbon dioxide in the air and it is customarily to prepare sodium hydroxide solution of approximate concentration and then standardize it against a primary standard to obtain its exact concentration. Potassium hydrogen phthalate is most commonly used to standardize sodium hydroxide solution as it's readily available in purity of 99.95%, nonhygroscopic, and with a high equivalent weight, 204.2g/mol.

The following equation can be used to denote reaction of titration:

$$\text{C}_6\text{H}_4(\text{COOH})(\text{COOK}) + \text{NaOH} \rightleftharpoons \text{C}_6\text{H}_4(\text{COONa})(\text{COOK}) + \text{H}_2\text{O}$$

The following equation can be used for calculation:

$$C_{\text{NaOH}} = \frac{w_{\text{KHC}_8\text{H}_4\text{O}_4}}{V_{\text{NaOH}} \cdot \frac{m_{\text{KHC}_8\text{H}_4\text{O}_4}}{1000}}$$

$$M_{\text{KHC}_8\text{H}_4\text{O}_4} = 204.2 \text{ (g/mol)}$$

Equipment

Burette (25mL), conical flask (250mL), volumetric cylinder (100mL), beaker (400mL), reagent bottle (500mL), rubber stopper.

Chemicals

Potassium hydrogen phthalate (primary standard), Sodium hydroxide (AR), Phenolphthalein indicator (0.1% alcoholic solution)

Procedures

Preparation of 0.1mol/L sodium hydroxide solution

Dissolve 2.2g of sodium hydroxide in the minimum amount of water, then transfer it to a rubber-stoppered bottle and dilute it to 500mL.

Standardization of sodium hydroxide solution

Weigh accurately into three clean, numbered conical flask about 0.45g of potassium hydrogen phthalate (dried at 105—110℃) respectively. To each flask add 50mL of distilled water and shake the flask gently until the sample is dissolved. Add 2 drops of phenolphthalein to each flask. Titrate the solutions to the first permanent pink color, which should persist not less than thirty seconds or so.

Demonstration of laboratory report

Original record

1. The weight of potassium hydrogen phthalate:
(1) $W_1 = 14.6758, W_2 = 14.2200, \Delta W = 0.4558$.
(2) $W_2 = 14.2200, W_3 = 13.7639, \Delta W = 0.4561$.
(3) $W_3 = 13.7639, W_4 = 13.2877, \Delta W = 0.4762$.

2. The volume of NaOH solution:

NaOH final reading: ① 21.78mL; ② 21.78mL; ③ 22.77mL.
NaOH initial reading: ① 0.00mL; ② 0.00mL; ③ 0.00mL.

Laboratory report (demonstration)

Preparation and standardization of solution hydroxide solution (Table 3):

Table 3 Preparation and standardization of solution hydroxide solution

	1	2	3
the weight of deta of material and bottle			
the weight of deta of material and bottle			
the weight of deta of material (g)			
V_{NaOH} (mL)			
C_{NaOH} (mol/L)			
means (mol/L)			

Notes

1. Weigh sodium hydroxide in a flask instead of on a piece of paper.
2. Put a label on each reagent bottle with the name of the reagent, date of preparation, operator, concentration, etc.
3. Rinse the drop-burette with sodium hydroxide solution three times before filling the drop-burette with sodium hydroxide solution.
4. Get rid of air bubbles from the tip of the drop-burette if there is any.
5. Adjust liquid level to zero point before each titration.

Questions

1. Why is it important to rinse the drop-burette with sodium hydroxide 3 times before titration? Is it necessary to dry and rinse the beakers with primary standard solution before titration? Why?
2. Is it necessary to adjust for the volume of the water used to dissolve the standard substance to be accurately measured?
3. Can methyl orange be applied as an indicator in this titration?
4. Why is it necessary to adjust liquid level to zero point before each titration?

Hailiqian Taoerdahon

EXPERIMENT FIVE

The Usage of Depression of Freezing Point to Determine the Molecular Weight of Glucose

Objectives

1. Understand Raoult's Law.
2. Learn the cryoscopy technique to determine the molecular weight.

Principles

The freezing point is the temperature at which tile vapor pressure of a solution (or solvent) equals the vapor pressure of its pure solid phase solvent. When the vapor pressure of the solution is less than the solvent at the same temperature, the freezing point is lowering. In general, solution has a lower freezing point than does the pure solvent.

The freezing point is determined by the concentration of the solution and the properties of the solvent. And the lowering of the freezing point is proportional to the quanlify of dissolved material.

The amount of the depression is given by

$$\Delta T_f = K_f m \text{ (nonelectrolyte solution)}$$

or,

$$\Delta T_f = iK_f m \text{ (electrolyte solution)}$$

Here, ΔT_f denotes the amount of the depression; i denotes van't Hoff mole number; m denotes molality which means the moles of the solute divide by the quantity of the solvent (mol/kg or mol (solute) /1000g (solvent)). For example, if "a" gram of solute (a/M mol) is soluble in "A" gram of solvent, then the molality $m = \dfrac{1000a}{AM}$ (M is the molecular weight of the solute). Putting the formula of m above into Raoult's expressions,

There exists:

$$\Delta T_f = K_f \dfrac{1000a}{AM}$$

or,

$$\Delta T_f = iK_f \frac{1000a}{AM}$$

Here, K_f is mole cryoscopic constant, which is only determined by the property of the solvent, but does not depend on the property of the solute. So different solvent has different value of K_f.

Equipment

1. 1/10 graduated thermometer: read to the second decimal digit.
2. Thin stirring rod.
3. Test tube: fill in the liquid to be determined.
4. Air coated tube: determine the freezing point accurately.
5. Thick wall beaker: fill in some ice water to decrease the temperature.
6. Rubber plug.

Chemicals

Glucose, coarse salt, ice.

Procedures

Determine the freezing point of the glucose solution

1. Preparation: fill some pieces of ice and a small quantity of water into a thick walled beaker (the volume of these two substances is about 3/4 of the whole beaker). Then add proper amount of coarse salts to decrease the temperature.

2. Then weigh 0.46—0.5g of glucose on the balance, pack the glucose carefully to avoid dispersing.

3. Determine the freezing point.

Put the glucose into a completely dry determining tube. then add 5mL distilled water from the inner wall of the tube with transfer pipette, shaking slightly. (Be carefully not to splash the solution out). When the glucose has dissolved completely, fill in the plug including the thermometer and the thin stirring rod, and insert them into the ice bath. Now stir the ice water with thick stirring rod and stir the glucose solution with thin stirring rod slightly. Take care not to touch the wall of the tube and the thermometer during the stirring process, If not, the heat produced from friction will affect the result. In the temperature decreasing process, super-cooling phenomenon happens (Don't freeze at freezing point). But with the temperature going on decreasing to a certain degree, it increase quickly to reach a certain point and then keeps at this point stably. The point at this temperature is called freezing point. Read and record accurately through magnifying glass.

Repeat the above process again. The difference of the two readings should be no more than 0.02℃. Average the two values for calculating the freezing point.

Determine the freezing point of the pure solvent (water)

Discard the solution in the determining tube. Wash the tube with tap water and then rinse it with distiller water. After adding 5mL distilled water, determine the freezing point of the water using the same method mentioned in operation 1.

Data record and result dealing

(1) Calculate the molecular weight of the glucose according to the result.

(2) Compare the result with the theoretical value.

(3) Data record and result dealing (Table 4).

Table 4 Data record and result dealing

experiment number	freezing point ℃		solute/g	solvent/g	ΔT_f
	distilled water	glucose solution			
1					
2					
3					
result: $M = iK_f \dfrac{1000a}{A\Delta T_f}$					

Instructions

Requirements

(1) Reason the concept of the freezing point. Tell the difference between the freezing points of pure solvent and the solution.

(2) Why the freezing point of solution is lower than that of pure solvent? Which law obeys the amount of depression of a dilute solution?

(3) Why could the ice in salt solution be used to decrease the temperature? If only ice water is used, what's the result?

(4) Why the freezing point of the pure solvent should be determined in this experiment?

(5) Can the cryoscopy technique be used to determine the molecular weight of a volatile substance?

Operation

(1) Learn to use the transfer pipette.

(2) Learn to record the temperature value from 1/10 graduated thermometer

(3) Determine the freezing point of a liquid.

Notes

(1) The determining tube should be dry.

(2) Notice that not to splash the quantitative solvent out of the determining tube.

(3) Use the magnifying glass to read the temperature from the 1/10 graduated thermometer.

(4) The glass of the bulb at the front tip of the thermometer is too thin (to promote the sensitivity for temperature measuring). Be sure not to replace the stirring rod with thermometer

(5) When determining the freezing point of the pure water, the thermometer may be frozen with ice. Notice to make the ice melt before taking it out.

(6) After determining the freezing point of tile solution and before determining the freezing point of the pure water, the determining tube should be washed carefully.

Report format

(1) Objectives.

(2) Principles.

(3) Data record and calculation.

Questions

Compare the experiment result with the theoretical value. Analyze the reason for error if any.

Hailiqian Taoerdahon

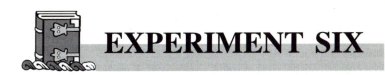

EXPERIMENT SIX

Determining the Ionization Constant of a Weak Acid

Objectives

1. To understand the concept of the ionization equilibrium.

2. To learn how to determine the ionization constant of a weak acid by pH-electrode potential measurement.

Principles

Acetic acid is a monobasic weak acid. An ionization equilibrium in aqueous solution can be represented by

$$HAc \rightleftharpoons H^+ + Ac^-$$

Hence the ionization constant is generally written as:

$$K_{HAc} = \frac{[H^+][Ac^-]}{[HAc]}$$

Take the logarithm of above formation:

$$\lg K_{HAc} = \lg[H^+] + \lg\frac{[Ac^-]}{[HAc]}$$

When $[Ac^-] = [HAc]$, there exists:

$$\lg K_{HAc} = \lg[H^+] + \lg 1 = \lg[H^+]$$

$$\lg K_{HAc} = \lg[H^+] = -pH$$

If the pH value of an acetic acid solution in which the concentration of $[HAc]$ equals to the concentration of $[Ac^-]$ is measured at a certain temperature, The approximate value of the ionization constant of acetic acid can be calculated.

Titrate HAc solution with NaOH. According to the reaction equation:

$$HAc + OH^- \rightleftharpoons Ac^- + H_2O$$

When $[HAc] = [Ac^-]$, the needed amount of NaOH should be equal to the half amount of NaOH when NaOH neutralizes HAc completely. If the pH value at this point is measured, then we can get the approximation of the ionization constant of acetic acid.

Equipment

(1) pH meter.

(2) Electrode.

(3) Two 100mL beakers, two 250mL Erlenmeyer flasks, 25mL acidic burette, 25mL basic burette.

Chemicals

NaOH 0.1mol/L standard solution; HAc about 0.1mol/L; buffer solution pH = 6.8—7; phenolphthalein indicator(1% ethanol solution).

Procedures

1. Transfer 22.00mL 0.1mol/L HAc from an acidic burette to a 250mL Erlenmeyer flask. Then add 2 drops of phenolphthalein solution. Titrate with 0.1mol/LNaOH standard solution. Shak constantly until the red color appears. Record the volume of NaOH added at the end point. Repeat the titration again in another Erlenmeyer flask. The difference between the volumes added in each titration should be no more than 0.10mL.

2. Transfer 22.00mL 0.1mol/L HAc from an acidic burette to a 100mL beaker. Titrate with 0.1mol NaOH standard solution until the volume of NaOH added is about the half of that added in operation 1 mentioned above. Stir constantly. Measure the pH value with pH meter.

3. Prepare the buffer solution:

(1) 0.025mol/L mixed phosphate solution (pH = 6.8—7.0). Weigh 3.53g Na_2HPO_4 and 3.39g KH_2PO_4 after each of them was dryed at 115℃ ±5℃ temperature. Then dissolve them with distilled water. Dilute to 1000mL in the volumetric flask.

(2) Saturated potassium tartrate solution(pH = 3.56). Mix an amount of distilled water and excessive hydrogen potassium tartrate powder in a glass bottle. Shake hard for about 20—30min. When the solution turns transparent and clean, take it for the next step with tilt-pour process.

4. Data record and result dealing: the concentration of the standard NaOH solution, mol/L _____.

The volume of HAc, mL (1)_____(2)_____.
The volume of NaOH added, mL (1)_____(2)_____.
The average volume of NaOH added, mL _____.

The pH value measured by pH meter _____.

According to the formation $\lg K_{HAc} = -pH$, calculate K_{HAc}_____.

Instruction

Requirement

(1) What principle does this experiment follow?

(2) When tile half amount HAc was neutralized by NaOH, It can be approximately considered to be $[HAc] = [Ac^-]$ in the solution, why?

(3) Will the value of pH be equal to 7.0 at the end point when HAc is neutralized by NaOH completely?

(4) Please list the key operation steps on measuring the pH value with pH meter.

Operation

(1) Learn to use pH meter correctly.

(2) Go on practicing the operation of titration and the burette's usage.

Notes

(1) The main sensible part of a glass electrode is a glass bulb in its upper part. The bulb is too thin, so be sure not to touch it with any hard substance. When the bulb is broken, this glass electrode will be invalid completely. Please notice to fix the glass bulb a little higher than the bottom part of the calomel electrode to avoid it being broken by the beaker.

A new glass electrode should be dipped into distilled water no less than 24 hours before being used or after being used.

But a compound electrode should be coated with a plastic cup containing 3mol/L KCl solution.

(2) The apparatus should be standardized by a standard buffer solution which has almost same pH value with the solution to be determined.

(3) Read the data twice or three times for determining each sample.

(4) After the experiment, rinse the electrodes with distilled water then reserve electrodes correctly.

Report Format

(1) Objectives.

(2) Principles.

(3) Data record and result dealing (Table 5).

Table 5 Data record and result dealing

	1	2
V_{HAc}/mL		
V_{NaOH}/mL		
V_{aNaOH}/mL		
the value of pH		

Questions

In this experiment we use pH-electrode potential to determine the ionization constant of acetic acid.

Chang Junmin

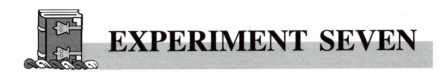

EXPERIMENT SEVEN

Buffer Solution

Objectives

1. Know the ionization equilibrium of weak acids, weak bases and principle of the shift of the equilibrium.

2. Practice how to prepare buffer solution and test its properties.

Principles

1. The ionization equilibrium of weak electrolytes and its shifting.

A weak electrolyte dissociates to a lesser extent when one of its ions is present in solution. For example, if sodium acetate, a strong electrolyte, is added to the acetic acid solution, the equilibrium will shift in the direction of forming acetic acid. It is called the common ion effect which makes the degree of ionization decreasing and the acidity of acetic acid decreasing.

2. Buffer solution: common ion effect has application in preparation of buffer solution. If add NaAc to HAc solution or add NH_4Cl to $NH_3 \cdot H_2O$, the concentration of $[H^+]$ and $[OH^-]$ change a little even if some: other acids or bases are added. This kind of solution consisting of a weak acid or a weak base-and its salt is named buffer solution.

Equipment

Acidometer, transfer pipette, burette.

Chemicals

Acid: HAc 1mol/L, 0.1mol/L; HCl 6mol/L, 0.1mol/L; citric acid 0.1mol/L.
Base: $NH_3 \cdot H_2O$ 2mol/L; 0.1mol/L, 6mol/L; NaOH 0.1mol/L.
Solid: NH_4Cl.
Salt: $MgCl_2$ 0.1mol/L, Na_3PO_4 0.1mol/L; NH_4Cl saturated solution 0.1mol/L. $CaCl_2$ 0.1mol/L; NaAc 0.5mol/L.

Other: phenolphthalein indicator, methyl orange indicator, thymol blue indicator.

Procedures

1. The ionization equilibrium of weak bases and the shift of the equilibrium (common ion effect).

(1) Take two test tubes, then add ln-1 distilled water, 2 drops-of 2mol/L $NH_3 \cdot H_2O$ and 1 drop of phenolphthalein indicator to each tube. Shake them and observe the color of the solutions. Then add a little amount of solid NH_4Cl to one tube. Please compare it with the other tube without NH_4Cl. Explain the reason of change.

(2) Add 2mL 2mol/L HAc solution to a test tube. Observe the color of the solution when 1 drop of methyl orange indicator is added. Then add a little amount of solid NaAc to it. What color: appears? Please draw a conclusion from that change.

(3) Take two tubes containing 5 drops of $MgCl_2$ solution. Add 5 drops of saturated NH_4Cl solution to one tube. Then add 5 drops of 2mol/L $NH_3 \cdot H_2O$ to each tube. Observe the different at phenomena in these two tubes.

2. Buffer solution:

(1) Add 3mL 0.1mol/L HAc and 3mL 0.1mol/L NaAc to a test-tube to prepare a buffer solution HAc-NaAc. Mix 5 drops of thymol blue indicator with it. Observe the color of the solution. Then divide the solution into three tubes (a, b and c). Add 5 drops of 0.1mol/L HCl to tube a, add 5 drops of 0.1mol/L NaAc to tube b, add 5 drops of H_2O to tube c. Observe the color change. Then add excessive amount of 0.1mol/L HCl to tube a, add excessive amount of 0.1mol/L NaOH to tube b, Pay attention to the color change. Then compare with the color in tube c. Please draw a conclusion from above.

The range of the color change of thymol blue indicator is as follows (Table 6):

Table 6 Buffer solution

tubes No.	pH	color
a	less than 2:8	red
b	8—9.6	yellow
c	more than 9.6	blue

(2) Prepare the buffer solution and observe the range of the color change of the indicator. Prepare the buffer solutions (pH = 2.2—5.0) according to the data shown in the table below (Table 7):

Table 7 Prepare the buffer solution

pH	0.1mol/L citric acid solution, mL	0.2mol/L Na_2HPO_4 solution, mL
2.2	19.60	0.40

Continued

pH	0.1mol/L citric acid solution, mL	0.2mol/L Na$_2$HPO$_4$ solution, mL
3.0	15.89	4.11
4.0	12.29	7.71
4.4	11.29	8.71
5.0	9.70	1030

Add 4mL of the prepared buffer solutions mentioned above to five test tubes respectively. Line up these tubes according to the sequence with the value of pH increasing. Then add one drop of methyl orange indicator to each tube. Observe the color change after shaking and tell the range of the color change of methyl orange (The range of color change of methyl orange is pH:3.0—4.4, red→orange).

(3) The property of the buffer solution. Take 25mL 0.1mol/L NH$_3 \cdot$ H$_2$O and 25mL 0.1mol/L NH$_4$Cl with transfer pipette to prepare a buffer solution. Determine the value of pH with acidometer (compare the determined value with the calculated value).

Add 0.5mL 0.1mol/L HCl (about 10 drops) to the buffer solution above, and determine the value of pH with acidometer. Then add 1mL 0.1mol/L NaOH (about 20 drops) and determine the value of pH (Table 8).

Table 8 The property of the buffer solution

buffer solution	determined pH value	calculated pH value
25mL 0.1mol/L NH$_3 \cdot$ H$_2$O		
25mL 0.1mol/L NH$_4$Cl		
add 0.5mL 0.1mol/L HCl		
add 1mL 0.1mol/L NaOH		

Instructions

Requirements

(1) What is common ion effect? Which experiment can test the common ion effect?

(2) To prepare a concentrated S^{2-} solution; which aqueous solution will you choose, H$_2$S or Na$_2$S? If only H$_2$S aqueous solution is offered, how to increase the concentration of S^{2-}?

(3) What is buffer solution? What properties does the buffer solution have?

(4) In this experiment, buffer solution HAc-NaAc is made up of 3mL 0.1mol/L HAc and NaAc. Can you evaluate the value of pH of the buffer solution according to the ionization equilibrium constant of HAc?

Operation

(1) Practice to use the acidometer;

(2) Practice the operation of burette and transfer pipette;

Notes

(1) To prevent from pollution, the dropping board should be cleaned with water before used and pH test paper can't be taken with hands directly.

(2) Every student can prepare a buffer solution in the experiment of "The properties of the buffer solution". Then add 0.5mL 0.1mol/L HCl and NaOH respectively. Last, determine the value of pH of each sample.

Report format (Table 9)

(1) Objectives.
(2) Principles.
(3) Procedures.

Table 9 Report

procedure	phenomenon	principle	conclusion

Questions

(1) To prepare a buffer solution (pH = 3), which is the best choose in the following electrolytes and their salts?

①HCOOH $K_a = 1.77 \times 10^{-4}$; ②HAc $K_a = 1.76 \times 10^{-5}$; ③$NH_3 \cdot H_2O$ $K_b = 1.79 \times 10^{-5}$.

(2) The solutions in the same couple are in the same concentration, which has higher value of pH?

①NaAc, NaCN; ②$NaHCO_3$, Na_2CO_3

Sun Lian

EXPERIMENT EIGHT

pH Measurement of Liquid Drug Preparation with pH Meter

Objectives

Grasp the principle and method of pH measurements with pH meter.

Principles

Presently pH measurements by direct potential method usually constitutes electrochemical cell, with a glass electrode employed as the measuring electrode (cathode) and a saturated calomel electrode is used as the reference electrode (anode) and these two electrodes are immersed in the solution.

$(-)$ Ag, AgCl (s) |HCl (0.1 mol/L) |H$^+$ (x mol/L) ‖ KCl (saturated) |Hg$_2$Cl$_2$, Hg(+). The potential for the cell is:

$$E = E_+ - E_- = E_{SCE} - E_{glass}$$
$$= E_{SCE} - (K_{glass} - \frac{2.303RT}{F}\text{pH})$$
$$= K + 0.059\text{pH}(25\,^\circ\text{C})$$

The above formula shows that the cell potential (E) is linear with the pH of the solution. Because the slope is $\frac{2.303RT}{F}$, and changes with the temperature, thus there is temperature-adjusting knob on pH meter to adjust with the temperature. In the practice, as the asymmetry potential will affect the K value and it is difficult to obtain accurately, the method of twice measurements is commonly used when measuring pH value with pH meter. First calibrate the pH meter against a standard buffer solution (which is called "orientation")

$$E_S = K + \frac{2.303RT}{F}\text{pH}_S$$

$$E_X = K + \frac{2.303RT}{F}\text{pH}_X$$

Subtract the two formula as each other and them:

$$E_s - E_x = \frac{2.303RT}{F}(pH_s - pH_x)$$

$$pH_x = pH_s + \frac{E_s - E_x}{2.303RT/F}$$

In order to reduce the deviation caused by the residue liquid junction potential on calibrating, pH of the selected buffer solution should be close to pH of the solution. The capability of some glass electrode or pH meter may have limitation, the calibration should be done by two buffers with different pH before measuring the solution pH. After orientated by one buffer solution, the other buffer solution, which pH value is 3 pH units different from the first buffer solution, the measuring error should be within ±0.1pH.

With the pH meter which has been orientated, pH value of the solution can be determined.

Equipment

pH meter, plastic beaker or glass beaker(25—50mL).

Chemicals

Potassium hydrogen phthalate standard buffer solution (0.05mol/L)
Mixed phosphate standard buffer solution
Glucose solution for injection
Physiological saline solution

Procedures

1. Install and manipulate the pH meter according to the operating rules on the manual (refer to the direction for use of the pH meter in Analytical Chemistry).

2. Experimental measurements.

Calibration: after orientate the pH meter by potassium hydrogen phthalate standard buffer solution, measure the pH value of the mixed phosphate standard buffer solution, compare with the oretical value.

Measurements: with the pH meter orientated above, measure the pH value of the glucose solution and the physiological saline, record the measured pH value for three times.

3. After finished the measurements. Clean the electrode and the beaker, repristinate the apparatus and turn off the power.

Notes

1. The glass ball at the lower end of the glass electrode is very thin, be sure not to touch the hard materials. The plug and the jack of the electrode should be keep clear, dry, dustproff, waterproof and anticorrosive.

2. Before use the glass electrode, the glass ball should be immersed in the distilled water at least one day. If keep warm in 50℃ distilled water for 2h, after cooled down to the room temperature, it can be used the very day. The glass ball is better to immerse in the distilled water for the next time usage.

3. When measuring the alkaline solution with glass electrode, do as quick as possible. As to measure the pH >9.0 solution, the high alkali glass electrode should be used.

4. On install the electrode, the end of the glass electrode should be 2—3mm higher than the saturated calomel electrode to avoid the glass electrode destroyed by touching the bottom of the beaker. There also should have a liquid level difference between the liquid level of KCl solution in the calomel electrode and the liquid level of the solution to be measured, to avoid diffuse into the calomel electrode. The special tip at the end of the tube should be covered by the rubber cover when the calomel electrode is not in use and do not allow the saturated KCl solution becomes air-dried.

5. The pH of the selected standard buffer solution for calibrate the pH meter should be close to the pH value of the solution to be measured ($\Delta pH \leqslant 3$). The temperature difference of the two solutions should be low than 1 ℃. The standard solution is better to be prepared by single alkaline salt or acidic salt. The reagents used should have high purity. Alkaline salt (such as sodium borate) is easy to efflorescence and absorb CO_2 in the air, it needs to be recrystalized before use. As for the pH meter the precision is 0.01, the sodium borate should be kept in humide state (70% humidity) made by saturated NaCl saccharose solution. The water for prepare the buffer solution is better to be the freshly boiled water after cooled down. The buffer solution is better to be kept in the polyethylene plastic bottle and sealed by wax if the lid is not very tightened.

6. When measure the pH value of weak buffer solution (such as H_2O) after calibration by selected potassium hydrogen phthalate standard buffer solution, measure the pH of the sample solution and the fresh sample solution again till the difference of the two data within 1min is not more than 0.05 pH. Then calibrate the pH meter by sodium borate standard buffer solution again and repeat to measure the pH value of the sample solution twice, the difference of the two data should be in the ranpe of ±0.1pH.

The average of the two data is the pH value of the sample solution.

7. After finish using the pH meter, the power should be turn off, the measurement range selector should be turn to "0", and the apparatus should be put in the dry environment and avoid the invasion of dust and corrosive gas.

Questions

1. Why should the pH meter be calibrated by the standard buffer solution with pH close to the pH value of the solution to be measured?

2. What should we pay attention to install the electrode?

Chang Junmin

EXPERIMENT NINE

Precipitation Equilibrium

Objectives

1. Understand the precipitation equilibrium and the shift of the equilibrium.
2. On the rule of the solubility product, please judge:
(1) The formation and dissolution of the precipitates.
(2) Transform of the precipitates and fractional precipitation.
3. Determine the value of the solubility product.

Principles

1. In the saturated solution of some slightly soluble salts, there is an equilibrium between the insoluble solid phase and part of the solid dissolving to form ions. Here, AB denotes slightly soluble salt, A^+ and B^- denote ions that are formed after part of AB dissolving. It exists in equilibrium as follows:

$$AB(s) \rightleftharpoons A^+ + B^- (aqueous)$$

With the formation of the precipitates, most of the relative ions can be separated from the solution, but it is impossible to remove all the ions.

In the above equilibrium, if the concentration of $[A^+]$ or $[B^-]$ is increased, the equilibrium shifts to the formation of precipitate AB. This is called "common ion effect".

Solubility product can be regarded as the standard rule to judge the formation or dissolution of precipitates. When $[A^+][B^-] > K_{sp}$, the precipitate is forming; when $[A^+][B^-] = K_{sp}$, the solution just turns to be saturated, while the precipitate is not forming yet; when $[A^+][B^-] < K_{sp}$, the solution is unsaturated no precipitate appears.

K_{sp} of some relative slightly soluble electrolytes are listed is table 10:

Table 10 K_{sp} of some relative slightly soluble electrolytes

slightly soluble electrolyte	Pb(SCN)$_2$	PbCl$_2$	PbI$_2$	PbCrO$_4$	CuS	PbS	Ag$_2$CrO$_4$
K_{sp}	2×10^{-5}	1.6×10^{-6}	7.1×10^{-9}	1.8×10^{-14}	1.3×10^{-36}	8.8×10^{-29}	1.1×10^{-12}

2. The molecule structure formula of thioacetamide is $CH_3\overset{\underset{\parallel}{S}}{C}\text{---}NH_2$.
It hydrolyzes to form H_2S to react with precipitate $PbCl_2$:

$$CH_3CSNH_2 + 2H_2O \rightleftharpoons CH_3COONH_4 + H_2S$$
$$PbCl_2 \downarrow \rightleftharpoons 2Cl^- + Pb^{2+}$$
$$H_2S \rightleftharpoons 2H^+ + S^{2-}$$
$$Pb^{2+} + S^{2-} \longrightarrow PbS \downarrow (\text{black})$$

3. If there are two kinds or more than two kinds of ions which can react with a precipitating reagent to form slightly soluble salts, the sequence of the formation of precipitation is dependent on the needed concentration of the precipitating reagent ions. The lowest concentration of the ion needed means precipitate will form at first, then another precipitate will form with the greater concentration of the ion needed. This known as fractional precipitation.

The process of transforming a slightly soluble electrolyte to another is called precipitate transform. As a common fact, the slightly soluble electrolyte with higher solubility can easily be transformed to those with lower value in solubility.

Equipment

Centrifuge, beaker.

Chemicals

Acid: HNO_3 6mol/L.

Base: NaOH 0.2mol/L; $NH_3 \cdot H_2O$ 2mol/L.

Salts: $Pb(NO_3)_2$ 0.1mol/L, 0.001mol/L; KI 0.1mol/L, 0.001mol/L; NH_4Cl 1mol/L; NH_4CNS 0.5mol/L; $FeCl_3$ 0.1mol/L; K_2CrO_4; 0.1mol/L; Na_2S 0.1mol/L; Na_2CO_3 0.1mol/L; NaCl 0.1mol/L; $MgCl_2$; 0.2mol/L; $(NH_4)_2C_2O_4$ saturated solution.

$AgNO_3$ 0.1mol/L; $CuSO_4$ 0.1mol/L; $CaCl_2$ 0.1mol/L; $BaCl_2$ 0.3mol/L; thioacetamide solution.

Others: pH test paper, pH = 5.5—9.0.

Procedures

Precipitation equilibrium and common ion effect

1. Precipitation equilibrium. Add 0.5mol/L NH_4CNS solution to 10 drops of 0.1mol/L $Pb(NO_3)_2$ solution until precipitate is forming completely. Shaking the tube (Because $Pb(SCN)_2$ easily occurs over-saturated) rub the inner wall of the test tube with

a glass rod, also shake the tube tempestuously. Separate the precipitate on centrifuge. Then add 0.1mol/L K_2CrO_4 to the above centrifugal solution. What happens? Try to illustrate if there exists Pb^{2+} in the centrifugal solution after separating the precipitate.

2. Common ion effect: Add 1mL saturated PbI_2 solution to a test tube, then add 5 drops of 0.1mol/L KI solution. Shake the tube for a moment. What happens?

Explain the reason.

The application of the solubility product

1. Formation of the precipitates.

(1) Add 1mL 0.1mol/L $Pb(NO_3)_2$ solution to a test tube, then add 1mL 0.1mol/L KI solution. Observe whether there are precipitates forming? Explain the reason.

(2) Add 1mL 0.001mol/L $Pb(NO_3)_2$ solution to a test tube, then add 1mL 0.1mol/L KI solution. Observe whether there are precipitates forming? Explain the reason.

(3) Add 2 drops of 0.1mol/L Na_2S solution and 5 drops of 0.1mol/L K_2CrO_4 to a centrifugal tube. Dilute with 5mL distilled water. Then add 5 drops of 0.1mol/L $Pb(NO_3)_2$ solution, Observe the color of the precipitate first appears (black or yellow?) centrifuge. Then drop 0.1mol/L $Pb(NO_3)_2$ solution to the centrifugal solution above the precipitate. What happens? (Observe the color of the precipitate). Illustrate the phenomena on the value of the solubility product.

2. Dissolution of the precipitates.

(1) Mix 3 drops of saturated oxalate amine solution with 5 drops of 0.3mol/L $BaCl_2$ solution, white precipitate is forming; centrifuge and discard the solution. Add 6mol/L HCl solution to the precipitate. What happens? Write out the reaction equation.

(2) Mix 10 drops of 0.1mol/L NaCl solution with 10 drops of 0.1mol/L $AgNO_3$ solution. Centrifuge to the precipitate. Discard the solution. Then add 2mol/L $NH_3 \cdot H_2O$ to the precipitate. What happens? Write out the reaction equation.

(3) Mix 5 drops of 0.2mol/L NaOH solution with 5 drops of 0.1mol/L $FeCl_3$ solution to form precipitate $Fe(OH)_3$; In another tube, mix 5 drops of 0.1mol/L Na_2CO_3 with 5 drops of 0.1mol/L $FeCl_3$ solution to form precipitate $CaCO_3$. Add 6mol/L HCl drop by drop to each precipitate mentioned above. What happens? Write out the reaction equation.

(4) Add 2mol/L $NH_3 H_2O$ drop by drop to a test tube containing 10 drops of 0.2mol/L $MgCl_2$ solution. Then with the addition of 1mol/L NH_4Cl solution, what happens? Write out the reaction equation.

(5) Add 5 drops of 0.1mol/L Na_2S solution to a test tube containing 5 drops of 0.1mol/L $CuSO_4$ solution. What happens? Then add 10 drops of 6mol/L HNO_3 solution

and heat slightly. What happens then? Write out the reaction equation.

3. Precipitate transform.

(1) Add 3 drops of 0.1mol/L NaCl solution to 5 drops of 0.1mol/L $Pb(NO_3)_2$ solution, white precipitate is forming. Then add 5 drops of thioacetamide solution and heat it over water bath. What happens? Explain the reason.

(2) Add 10 drops of 0.1mol/L K_2CrO_4 solution to 10 drops of 0.1mol/L $AgNO_3$ solution. Add to it 0.1mol/L, NaCl solution, what happens? Write out the reaction equation.

Predict the value of the solubility product of $Mg(OH)_2$

Add 25mL of 0.2mol/L $MgCl_2$ to a 50mL beaker underlaid a piece of black paper at the bottom. Then add 0.2mol/L NaOH solution to $MgCl_2$ solution drop by drop. Stir constantly until precipitate is forming. (Please observe on the blazing sunshine directly). Notice that NaOH solution added should not be excessive. (Why?) Determine the value of pH of the solution with pH test paper. Calculate $[OH^-]$ and K_{sp}.

Instructions

Requirements

(1) Point out the different and the common properties between the slightly soluble electrolyte and the weak electrolyte. Notice to distinguish the concepts of degree of ionization "solubility".

(2) Point out the common points between the precipitation equilibrium and the ionization equilibrium.

(3) Is the common ion effect in the precipitation equilibrium same as that in the ionization equilibrium?

(4) What is the condition of the precipitate formation?

(5) What is fractional precipitation? How to judge about the sequence of the formation of the precipitates in a certain experiment on the value of the solubility product?

(6) Please list several methods of dissolving the precipitates.

(7) What should be noticed on writing the precipitation reaction equation?

(8) Among the following substances, which will be precipitated from the water?

$Pb(Ac)_2$, $Pb(SCN)_2$, $Pb(NO_3)_2$, $PbCrO_4$, PbI_2, $BaCl_2$, BaC_2O_4, $AgCl$, $[Ag(NH_3)_2]Cl$, Ag_2CrO_4, $FeCl_3$, $Fe(OH)_3$, $CaCO_3$, Na_2CO_3, $Mg(OH)_2$, $CuSO_4$, CuS.

(9) Explain the precipitate transform by comparing the K_{sp} of $PbCl_2$, $PbSO_4$, $PbCrO_4$, PbS?

Operation

(1) Learn to use centrifuge.

(2) Practice to heat over the water bath.

Notes

1. How to use the centrifuge.

(1) Remember the centrifuge tube place.

(2) Centrifuge tube should be placed symmetrically to prevent the friction caused by unbalanced weigh. When a solution is to be centrifuged, another empty tube should be added with the same volume of distilled water and be placed symmetrically to balance in centrifuge.

(3) When finishing the separation, please don't stop the axis of the centrifuge by your hand but allow it stop naturally.

2. How to separate the precipitate from the solution

Pinch the rubber part of a capillary tube, then insert it into a test tube. Be sure that the tip of the capillary tube is near the surface of the precipitate but not touch it. Then loosen the rubber part, transfer the absorbed solution from the precipitate. Repeat several times to transfer the solution as possible as you can.

3. Heating over water bath is a kind of method when the sample should be heated for a long time at a certain range of temperature, There are also air bath, sand bath and vapor bath. Water bath can be in a copper boiler or in a beaker (Heat some water in a beaker, then put the sample that need to be heated into the beaker).

4. Centrifugal tube is marked with graduation. Its bottom part is too thin, Because the thickness of the whole tube is not well-proportioned, it can't be heated directly on fire, but only in the water bath.

Report format

(1) Objectives.

(2) Procedures.

Conclusion: there exists Pb^{2+} ion in the solution after separation.

Questions

1. How do the reaction conditions (such as temperature and concentration) affect the spontaneouely of the precipitation reaction?

2. How to get $Pb(Ac)_2$ from $PbCl_2$ solution consisting of Fe^{2+}, Cu^{2+}?

Chang Junmin

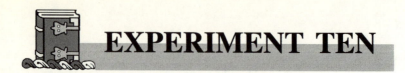

EXPERIMENT TEN

Redox Reaction

Objectives

1. To explain the intrinsic properties of redox reaction, and acquainte with some common oxidizing and reducing agents.

2. To learn about some metals location in the table of electrode potentials, and enhance the knowledge about electrode potentials.

3. To compare the relative strengths of reducing and oxidizing agents.

4. To learn about the influence of concentration, acidity and temperature on redox reaction.

5. To learn to assemble a galvanic cell and electrolysis with the galvanic cell.

Principles

A very large class of reactions can be regard as occurring by loss of electrons from one substance and gain by another substance. Since electron gain is known as reduction and electron loss as oxidation, the joint process is considered to be an oxidation reduction reaction, or more simply, redox reaction. The substance that supplies electrons (the oxidation number of an atom decreases) is the reducing agent and the substance that gains electrons (the oxidation number of an atom increases) is the oxidizing agent. The reducing agent is to be oxidized while the oxidizing agent is to be reduced. Oxidation and reduction always occur together, and the number of electrons gained by the oxidizing agent must be identical to the number of electrons lost by the reducing agent.

Electrode potentials can be applied to judge the relative intensity of oxidezing and reducing agents and determine the potential direction of a given redox reaction. The concentration, pH and temperature have effects on magnitude of the electrode potential. The table of standard electrode potentials can be used as the summary of the redox reaction rules in aqueous solution. In the table of standard electrode potentials, generally, the reducing agent (written at the right side of the reactions) in the upper part of the table is stronger reducing agent, which reduces the oxidizing agents below it. Conversely, the oxidizing agent (written at left side of the reactions) in the bottom of the table is stronger oxidizing agent, which oxides the reducing agents above it.

A galvanic cell is a device designed to produce electron current based on redox reactions.

Na_2SO_4 solution can be electrolyzed with the electron current produced by a galvanic cell.

Equipment

Tube, beaker.

Chemicals

Solid: granulated plumbum; granulated zinc

Acid: HNO_3 (2mol/L, conc.); HCl 1mol/L; H_2SO_4 (3mol/L, 1mol/L); HAc 6mol/L; H_2S solution.

Alkili: NaOH (40%, 6mol/L)

Salt: $KMnO_4$ 0.01mol/L; $FeSO_4$ 0.5mol/L; Na_2SO_3 0.1mol/L; $Na_2C_2O_4$ 0.1mol/L; NaBr 1mol/L; $K_2Cr_2O_7$ 0.1mol/L; NaI 1mol/L; $Fe_2(SO_4)_3$ 0.025mol/L; $Pb(NO_3)_2$ 1mol/L, $CuSO_4$ 1mol/L; Na_2SO_4 0.5mol/L; $MnSO_4$ 0.2mol/L; $AgNO_3$ 0.1mol/L.

Others: litmus test paper (red); H_2O_2 3%; $CHCl_3$

Procedures

Oxidizing agents and reducing agents

1. Mix 5 drops of 0.01mol/L $KMnO_4$ solution with 3 drops of H_2SO_4 (3mol/L) solution in each of two tubes. To one tube add 1—2 drops of H_2O_2 (3%), and to another tube add 2—3 drops of $FeSO_4$ (0.5mol/L) solution. Observe the reactions and point out the oxidizing agents and reducing agents,

$$KMnO_4 + H_2SO_4 + H_2O_2 \longrightarrow MnSO_4 + O_2 \uparrow + K_2SO_4 + H_2O$$
$$KMnO_4 + H_2SO_4 + FeSO_4 \longrightarrow MnSO_4 + Fa_2(SO_4)_3 + K_2SO_4 + H_2O$$

2. Add 3 drops of 0.1mol/L $K_2Cr_2O_7$ solution to 5 drops of 3mol/L H_2SO_4 solution, then add a few drops of H_2S solution. Observe the reaction and point out the oxidizing agent and reducing agent.

$$K_2Cr_2O_7 + H_2SO_4 + H_2S \longrightarrow Cr_2(SO_4)_3 + S \downarrow + KHSO_4 + H_2 \uparrow$$

Locate the sequence of Zn, Pb, Cu in the table of electrode potentials

Mix granulated zinc with 3mL of 1mol/L $Pb(NO_3)_2$ and 1mol/L $CuSO_4$ solution respectively, and observe.

Mix granulated plumbum with 3mL of 1mol/L $ZnSO_4$ and $CuSO_4$ solution respectively, and observe.

Formulate the reaction equations, and locate the relative sequence of Zn, Cu, Pb in the table of electrode potentials. Explain the relation between the relative sequence and the activities of the metals.

Factors influencing redox reactions

1. The effect of concentration on redox reactions. Mix granulated zinc with 2mL concentrated HNO_3 and 2mol/L HNO_3 respectively. Observe the reactions, and point out the differences of reaction rates and products. The reduced product of concentrated HNO_3, NO_2, can be detected by its color, while the reduced product of diluted HNO_3 (NH_4^+) can be detected by the following test.

Detection of NH_4^+ (with a gas chamber): Place 5 drops of the detected solution and 3 drops of 6mol/L NaOH solution on a watch glass, cover the watch glass with another smaller watch glass, attaching beforehand a piece of moist red litmus paper on the concave side. Then observe the litmus paper in 10 minutes. The blue color of red litmus paper indicates the presence of the NH_4^+ ion in the solution.

2. The effect of pH on reaction rate. To two portions of 0.5ml of 1mol/L NaBr solution acidified with 10 drops of 3mol/L H_2SO_4 and 6mol/L HAc solution respectively, add 1 drop of 0.01mol/L $KMnO_4$ solution. Compare the rate of decolorization of both samples.

Write out the reaction equation, and explain the difference in reaction rate

3. The effect of temperature on reaction rate. Add 2mL of 0.1mol/L $Na_2C_2O_4$ solution, 0.5ml of 3mol/L H_2SO_4 solution and 1 drop of 0.01mol/L $KMnO_4$ solution into each of two tubes, shake and mix. Heat one tube in 80℃ water bath, while keep another tube under room temperature. Compare the rate of decolorization of both samples. Write out the reaction equation, and explain the difference between the two solutions.

4. The effect of pH on redox reaction products. Add 10 drops of 1mol/L H_2SO_4, distilled water, 40% NaOH solution respectively into three tubes containing 10 drops of 0.1mol/L Na_2SO_3. Shake and add 3 drops of 0.01mol/L $KMnO_4$ solution to the tubes. Observe the reactions and write out the reaction equations. In acid solution MnO_4^- is reduced to the pale pink manganous ion, Mn^{2+}. In neutral solution MnO_4^- is reduced to black, insoluble, solid MnO_2, although in strongly alkaline solution it can be reduced to the Mn +6 state, existing as the bright green manganate ion, MnO_4^{2-}.

The effect of catalyst on redox reactions

Mix 5mL of 0.2mol/L $MnSO_4$ solution and 1mL of 3mol/L H_2SO_4 solution, then add a spoon of solid $(NH_4)_2S_2O_8$. Shake constantly to dissolve the solid completely. Divide the solution into two portions. Add 1—2 drops of 0.1mol/L $AgNO_3$ solution to one portion, while add nothing to another. Observe and write out the reaction equation. Explain the difference of the two portions of solution.

Selection of oxidizing agents

Between the commonly used oxidizing agents, $Fe_2(SO_4)_3$ and $KMnO_4$, choose an oxidizing agent which can oxidize I^- into I_2 while not oxidize Br^- into Br_2 in the solution of NaBr and NaI. Tests:

(1) Add 10 drops of 3mol/L H_2SO_4, 1mL of $CHCl_3$ and 2—3 drops of 0.01mol/L $KMnO_4$ into each of two tubes containing 10 drops of 1mol/L NaBr solution and 10 drops of 1mol/L NaI solution. Mix by shaking constantly and observe the color of $CHCl_3$ layer in the two tubes.

The color of I_2 in $CHCl_3$ is pink (or purple), and Br_2 showing orange color.

(2) Substitute $KMnO_4$ solution with $Fe_2(SO_4)_3$ solution and repeat the same operation above, Observe the color of $CHCl_3$ layer in the two tubes.

Write out the reaction equations and select the appropriate oxidizing agent. Explain your selection.

Instruction

Requirements

(1) Write out the usual reduced products of the following oxidants and oxidized products of the following reductants.

Oxidants: MnO_4^- (in acidic medium), H_2O_2, CrO_4^{2-}, H_2SO_4 (conc), HNO_3 (2mol/L), MnO_4^- (in neutral medium), Fe^{3+}, Cu^{2+}, $S_2O_8^{2-}$, Cl_2, Br_2, MnO_4^-, (in alkaline medium), $Cr_2O_7^{2-}$, Pb^{4+}, HNO_3 (concentrated), I_2.

Reductants: $H_2O_2, Zn, Br^-, C_2O_4^{2-}, Fe^{2+}, S^{2-}, I^-, SO_3^{2-}$.

(2) Taking Zn, Pb, Cu as examples to explain how to judge on the basis of standard electrode potentials whether a displace reaction between metals can be carried out?

(3) What factors will affect the electrode potential?

(4) What are the influence of concentration and pH on the redox reaction products and directions?

(5) How to assemble a Cu-Zn galvanic cell? What is the use of the salt bridge?

(6) Why can not get solid sodium at the cathode during the electrolysis of Na_2SO_4

solution?

(7) Complete the following reactions.

$MnO_4^- + H_2O_2 + H^+ \longrightarrow$

$MnO_4^- + Fe^{2+} + H^+ \longrightarrow$

$Cr_2O_7^{2-} + H_2S + H^+ \longrightarrow$

$Zn + HNO_3(2mol/L) \longrightarrow$

$MnO_4^- + Br^- + H^+ \longrightarrow$

$MnO_4^- + C_2O_4^{2-} + H^+ \longrightarrow$

$MnO_4^- + S^{2-} + H^+ \longrightarrow$

$MnO_4^- + S^{2-} + H_2O \longrightarrow$

$MnO_4^- + S^{2-} + OH^- \longrightarrow$

$S_2O_8^{2-} + Mn^{2+} + H_2O \longrightarrow$

Operation

Master the method of detecting ammonium ion in a gas chamber.

Notes

(1) The reaction between concentrate HNO_3 and Zn will liberate poisonous gas, NO_2, and it should be carried out in a hood.

(2) Owing to the low reaction rates, in the test of locating the sequence of tubes should be placed in the test tube rack for a while without any disturbance.

Report format

(1) Objectives.
(2) Principle.
(3) Procedure (illustrated with tables).

Questions

(1) Can a conclusion being obtained on that a redox reaction consisting of two half-reactions will occur at a higher reaction rate to a larger ΔE^θ?

(2) How to use the table of electrode potentials to form a redox reaction equation?

(3) What conditions will be required for the table of electrode potentials be used to judge the direction of a given redox reaction? And under what conditions will the Nernst equation be used?

Sun Lian

EXPERIMENT ELEVEN

Determination of Solubility Product of AgAc

Objectives

To understand the principle and method of determining the solubility product of AgAc.

Principle

In the aqueous solution of an insoluble or slightly soluble electrolyte, there exists equilibrium between the ions and the insoluble solid. The equilibrium constant for the dissolution of an insoluble or slightly soluble electrolyte is called the solubility product.

In writing the equation for the equilibrium, it is convention to write as:

$$A_mB_n(s) \rightleftharpoons mA^{n+} + nB^{m-}$$

The equilibrium constant $K = [A^{n+}]^m [B^{m-}]^n / [A_mB_n]$

So we can get $K_{sp} = [A^{n+}]^m [B^{m-}]^n$, just as $[A_mB_n]$ is unchangeable in constant temperature.

Equipment

Erlenmeyer flask, burette, transfer pipette, beaker.

Chemicals

Acid: HNO_3　6mol/L.

Salt: $AgNO_3$　0.20mol/L; NH_4Ac　0.20mol/L; $Fe(NO_3)_3$ solution; standard solution of KSCN 0.1mol/L.

Procedures

1. Add 20mL of $AgNO_3$ solution and 40mL of NH_4Ac solution (0.2mol/L) with two burettes respectively to a dry Erlenmeyer flask marked 1, 30mL of $AgNO_3$ solution and 30mL of NH_4Ac solution (0.2mol/L) to another dry Erlenmeyer flask marked 2. The

volumes of solution in the two flasks are same to be 60mL. Shake the flasks constantly for about 30mins until the precipitates form completely. The solid and ions in solution are in balance.

Filter the solutions with dry filter paper to two dry beakers respectively (filter again if the filtrate is not clear). Transfer 25mL No. 1 filtrate with a transfer pipette to a clean Erlenmeyer flask, add 1mL of HNO_3 (6mol/L) and 1mL of $Fe(NO_3)_3$ solution (indicator) to the Erlenmeyer flask. Add more HNO_3 solution if the color of solution is red (causing by hydrolysis of ferric ion), until the solution is colorless. Titrate the solution with standard solution of KSCN. The end point is reached when the color of solution is unchangeable pale pink. Record the volume of the KSCN solution. Repeat the operation of titration with the same filtrate.

Titrate the filtrate in No. 2 beaker with the same method above.

$$AgNO_3 + NH_4Ac \rightleftharpoons AgAc \downarrow + NH_4NO_3$$
$$Ag^+ + SCN^- \rightleftharpoons AgSCN \downarrow$$
$$Fe^{3+} + 3SCN^- \rightleftharpoons Fe(SCN)_3$$

2. Data record and process.

(1) Data record Table 11:

Table 11 Data record

	1	2
The volume of $AgNO_3$ solution, mL		
The volume of NH_4Ac solution, mL		
The volume of the mixture, mL		
The volume of filtrate for titration, mL	(1)	(2)
	(2)	(1)
The concentration of KSCN solution, mol/L		

(2) Data process (Table 12):

Table 12 Data process

	1	2
$[Ag^+]$ in the mixture (including precipitated)		
$[Ac^-]$ in the mixture (including precipitated)		
$[Ag^+]$ in the filtrate (taking the average value of the two tests to the following calculation)		
$[Ag^+]$ the precipitated as AgAc	(1)	(2)
$[Ac^-]$ in the filtration	(2)	(1)
The solubility product $K_{sp} = [Ag^+][Ac^-]$		

EXPERIMENT ELEVEN · 45 ·

Instructions

Requirements

(1) Explain the concept of Ksp. Will the Ksp be kept as a constant on adding other soluble strong electrolytes to the solution of insoluble electrolyte?

(2) Explain the principle of this experiment in determining solubility product of AgAc.

(3) Why the volume of $AgNO_3$ and NH_4Ac solution should be transferred precisely?

(4) Why the mixture solution should be filter with dry filter paper?

(5) What glassware should be dried beforehand? And why?

(6) How to calculate the K_{sp} of AgAc from the experiment results? (All the calculation data should contain four significant figures.)

(7) Which figures in the chart can be. calculated in advance?

Operation

(1) To practice the operation of transferring solution with burettes and transfer pipette precisely.

(2) To learn about locating the end point of titration when the indicator is $Fe(SCN)_3$.

Notes

(1) The Erlenmeyer flasks, short-stem funnels, beakers and glass rod used in the experiment should be cleaned and dried in advance. The transfer pipette should be rinsed three times with the filtrate used in the pipette.

(2) The burettes for different solution should be labeled. The Erlenmeyer flasks and beakers should be marked with number.

(3) To ensure the AgAc to be precipitated completely and the solution not to be splashed out, special care should be taken in shaking the Erlenmeyer flasks?

(4) Dry filter papa should be used to filtrate the mixture. If the filter paper is not dry, the first 1—2mL filtration should be discharged.

(5) The color of solution should be reddish when the end point is reached.

(6) To prevent Ag from precipitating on the inner wall of the apparatus, the glassware should be wash instantly. The burette filled with $AgNO_3$ solution should be washed with distilled water instead of tapwater, otherwise AgCl will precipitated on the inner wall of the burette.

Report format

(1) Objectives.

(2) Principle.

(3) Data record and process(shown in charts).

Questions

(1) Compare the laboratory value of K_{sp} with 4.4×10^{-3}, the theoretical value, and explain the deviation.

(2) What are the effects on the experimental result of incomplete precipitation or penetration the filter paper of AgAc?

Yao Jun

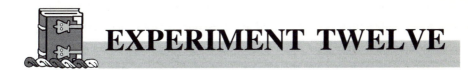

EXPERIMENT TWELVE

Determining the Coordination Number of $[Ag(NH_3)_n]^+$

Objectives

1. To determine the coordination number (n) of $[Ag(NH_3)_n]^+$ and to calculate its stability on the basis of coordination equilibrium principle and solubility product principle.

2. To be familiar with acidic burette and transfer pipette.

Principle

Excess ammonia water is added into silver nitrate solution and stable complex ion consisting of Ag^+ and NH_3 is obtained, then potassium bromide solution is added until the precipitation of silver bromide appear. At this time, the coordination equilibrium and precipitation equilibrium coexist in the mixture.

Coordination equilibrium

$$Ag^+ + nNH_3 = [Ag(NH_3)_n]^+$$

$$K_s = \frac{[Ag(NH_3)_n^+]}{[Ag^+][NH_3]^n} \tag{1}$$

Precipitation equilibrium

$$Ag^+ + Br^- = AgBr(s)$$

$$K_{sp} = [Ag^+][Br^-] \tag{2}$$

(1) × (2)

$$K = K_s \times K_{sp} = \frac{[Ag(NH_3)_n^+][Br^-]}{[NH_3]^n} \tag{3}$$

Then:

$$[Br^-] = \frac{K \times [NH_3]^n}{[Ag(NH_3)_n^+]} \tag{4}$$

$[Ag^+]$, $[Br^-]$ and $[Ag(NH_3)_n^+]$ represent the equilibrium concentrations and can be approximately by the following method:

If, in each portion of the mixture, the volume of silver nitrate solution we initially took V_{Ag^+} (same in each portion) and the concentration is $[A^+]_0$, if the volume of ammonia water (substantial excess) we added subsequently into each portion is V_{NH_3} and the concentration is $[NH_3]_0$, if the volume of potassium bromide solution we added subsequently into each Portion is V_{Br^-} and the concentration is $[Br^-]_0$, And If the total volume of mixture is V_t, then, when equilibrium is reached mixture, we have:

$$[Br^-] = [Br^-]_0 \times \frac{V_{Br}}{V_t} \qquad (5)$$

$$[Ag(NH_3)_n^+] = [Ag^+]_0 \times \frac{V_{Ag^+}}{V_t} \qquad (6)$$

$$[NH_3] = [NH_3]_0 \times \frac{V_{NH_3}}{V_t} \qquad (7)$$

Put (5), (6) and (7) into equation (4), then we have

$$V_{Br^-} = V_{NH_3}^n \times K \times \left[\frac{[NH_3]_0}{V_t}\right]^n \bigg/ \frac{[Br^-]_0}{V_t} \times \frac{[Ag^+]_0 \times V_{Ag^+}}{V_t} \qquad (8)$$

All except for in the right side of equation (8) are constants, so equation (8) can be transformed to:

$$V_{Br^-} = V_{NH_3}^n \times K' \qquad (9)$$

Draw the logarithms at both sides of the equation (9), we can obtain a linear equation:

$$\lg V_{Br^-} = n \lg V_{NH_3} + \lg K'$$

Make the graph (assign $\lg V_{Br^-}$ to Y-coordinate, $\lg V_{NH_3}$ to X-coordinate and $\lg K'$ to intercept) and then we can get the value of the slope (n) which is also the value of the coordination number of $[Ag(NH_3)_n^+]$ (take the closest integer).

Equipment

Transfer pipette (20mL); Erlenmeyer flask (250mL); graduated cylinder (100mL); two burettes.

Chemicals

Silver nitrate (0.01mol/L); potassium bromide (0.01mol/L); ammonia (2mol/L).

Procedures

Operation

Transferring pipette should be used to transfer 0.01mol/L silver nitrate solution of 20.00mL into a 250mL Erlenmeyer flask, then 40.00mL 2.0mol/L ammonia water is added through the basic burette and distilled water of 40mL is added by the graduation cylinder into Erlenmeyer flask. And then, stirring continuously, 0.01mol/L potassium bromide solution should be added though the acidic burette drop until the precipitate of silver bromide can't disappear, then stop titration and write down the volume (V_{Br^-}) of potassium bromide solution which has been used and the total volume (V_t) of the solution in that flask. The above procedure is repeated by adding water of different volume respectively (35mL, 30mL, 25mL, 20mL, 15mL and 10mL). In order to keep V_t in every repeated experiment the volume as that of fast experiment, some distilled water must be added when the endpoint is close.

Records and Data

(1) Records:

(2) Data:

(a) Please draw the graph with $\lg V_{Br^-}$, assigned to Y-coordinate and $\lg V_{NH_3}$ assigned to X-coordinate.

(b) Get the value of n from the graph and calculate the value of K from Equation (10).

(c) Calculate the value of K from Equation (8).

(d) On the basis of the equation: $K = K_{sp,AgBr} K_s$, we can finally get the value of K_s. (reference value: $K_{sp,AgBr} = 4.1 \times 10^{-13}$)

Instructions

Requirement

(1) What is K_s? By which method can K_s of $[Ag(NH_3)_n]^+$ and its coordination number be determined?

(2) How can coordination equilibrium and precipitation equilibrium coexist?

(3) The used Erlenmeyer flasks in this experiment must be clean and dry at the beginning, and cannot be washed with water during titration. What is and redurence between this experiment and Acid-Base titration experiment? Arid why?

Operation

(1) To grasp how to control the end point during titration.

(2) To learn techniques in data processing and graph making.

Notes

(1) During-the won fox each mixture, ammonia water is added finally (lest ammonia would volatilize away).

(2) before the end point can be observed, an equilibrium state should be reached for the reaction, and the extent of turbidity for each end point should be the same.

(3) At last, pipets and Erlenmeyer flasks contaminated with silver nitrate should be washed with ammonia water left.

Report format

(1) Objective.

(2) Principle.

(3) Procedure.

(a) Record(see the table list above).

(b) Date process (see the demand above).

(c) Discussion (analyze the come of error).

Question

(1) Why should the following situation be ignored when the equilibrium concentration of (NH_3), $[Br^-]$ and $[Ag(NH_3)_n]^+$ calculated?

(a) The amount of Br^- and Ag^+ used to produce the precipitate of silver bromide

(b) The amount of Ag^+ dissociated from $[Ag(NH_3)_n]^+$

(c) The amount of ammonia used to produce the complex ion of $[Ag(NH)_n^+]$

(2) If excess potassium, bromide solution was added during titration, should solution in the Erlenmeyer flask be thrown away for a turn-over-a-new-leaf?

(3) Is V_{Br^-} always the same in every titration? and how about $[Br^-]$?

Yao Jun

EXPERIMENT THIRTEEN

Coordination Compounds

Objectives

To learn about the set of conditions to form coordination compounds and the application of coordination compounds.

Principles

The reactions of forming coordination compounds are reversible. For example:

$$Cu^{2+} + 4NH_3 = [Cu(NH_3)_4]$$

1. Increasing the concentration of ligand(NH_3) will cause a shift of the equilibrium to the side of complex ion. Conversely, decreasing the concentration of ligand will result in a reverse shift of the equilibrium.

2. Adding a precipitant to precipitate the central metal ion will destroy the complex ion. Adding a ligand, which reacts with the central metal ion to form stable complex ion, can dissolve the slightly soluble salts of the metal ion. To the solution of the metal ion, adequate ligands added prior to the precipitant will prevent the precipitation.

3. If the ligand is a weak base or the anion of weak acid, adding strong acid will destroy the complex ion.

4. Adding two kinds of ligands the solution of a metal ion, a more stable complex ion will be formed. For instance, adding Fe^{3+} to the solution of F^- and CN^-, we will get $[FeF_6]^{3-}$ instead of $[Fe(NCS)_6]^{3-}$.

5. The outer electron structure of the central metal ion will change by adding ligands to form complex ion. Consequently its redox property will change also. A instance is that $[Co(CN)_6]^{4-}$ has stronger reductive ability than Co^{2+}.

6. By adding excess $NH_3 \cdot H_2O$ to the complex ion of Cr^{3+} and EDTA, $[Cr(OH)Y]^{2-}$ will be formed.

7. There are some constants needed in this experiment:

$$K_{sp, AgCl} = 1.8 \times 10^{-10}$$

$$K_{sp,AgBr} = 5.3 \times 10^{-13}$$
$$K_{sp,AgI} = 8.5 \times 10^{-17}$$
$$K_{s[Ag(NH_3)_2]} = 1.5 \times 10^7$$
$$K_{s[Ag(S_2O_3)_2]} = 2.4 \times 10^{13}$$
$$K_{s[Ag(CN)_2]} = 1.3 \times 10^{21}$$
$$E^{\ominus}_{CO^{3+}/CO^{2+}} = +1.842$$
$$E^{\ominus}_{I_2/I^-} = +0.5345$$

Equipment

Solid: $CuSO_4 \cdot 5H_2O$; NaF.

Acid: HCl 1mol/L.

Alkali: ammonium solution (2mol/L, conc.); NaOH 1mol/L; Na_2CO_3 0.1mol/L.

Salt: Na_2S 0.1mol/L; $BaCl_2$ 0.1mol/L; KSCN 1mol/L; NaCl 0.1mol/L; KBr 0.1mol/L; EDTA-2Na 0.1mol/L; $K_4P_2O_7$; $Na_2S_2O_3$ 0.5mol/L; KCN 0.5mol/L; $AgNO_3$ 0.1mol/L;

KI 0.1mol/L; Sodium citrate 1mol/L; $CuSO_4$ 0.1mol/L; $CaCl_2$ 0.1mol/L; $CoCl_2$ 0.5mol/L; $CrCl_3$ 0.1mol/L.

Other: ethanol(95%); H_2O_2(30%); starch solution; acetone; pH test paper or red litmus paper; phenolphthalein; iodine solution.

Procedure

Formation of coordination compounds

Preparation and properties of $[Cu(NH_3)_4]SO_4$

Reaction: $CuSO_4 + 4NH_3 \rightleftharpoons [Cu(NH_3)_4]SO_4$

Operation

Dissolve 2.5g $CuSO_4 \cdot 5H_2O$ (0.01mol) with 10mL of water in a beaker, add 5mL of concentrated ammonia solution (0.07mol), mix the solution, then add 15mL of ethanol and stir. Waiting 2—3 minutes, filter and collect the crystal of $[Cu(NH_3)_4]SO_4 \cdot H_2O$, wash the crystal with two portions of ethanol. Record the appearance of the crystal.

Property

(1) Dissolve a portion of the product in several drops of water, observe and record the color of the solution. Add more drops of water and observe the color change.

(2) Dissolve a portion of the product in several drops of water, add excess 1mol/L HCl solution drop by drop, observe and record the color change of the solution. Then

add excess concentrated ammonia solution to observe the color change. Discuss the formation and dissociation of $[Cu(NH_3)_4]SO_4$ in solution basing on the tests.

(3) Dissolve a portion of the product in several drops of water, divide the solution to three parts.

Add 0.1mol/L Na_2CO_3 solution to the first part, and observe whether there are $Cu(OH)_2CO_3$ precipitated from the solution.

Add 0.1mol/L Na_2S solution to the second part, and observe whether there are CuS precipitated from the solution.

Discuss the concentration change of Cu^{2+} in the two portions of solution basing on the tests above.

Add 0.1mol/L $BaCl_2$ solution to the third part, and observe whether there are $BaSO_4$ precipitated from the solution.

Discuss the function of Cu^{2+} and SO_4^{2-} in $[Cu(NH_3)_4]^{2+}$.

(4) Smell a portion of dried product to determine whether there is the odor of NH_3, then put it in a dry test tube, and hang a piece of moisten pH paper or red litmus paper near the opening of the tube and heat the crystal. Observe and record: ①the color change of the test paper, ②the color of the residue in the tube, ③the odor appearing in the tube. Write out the reaction equation.

Conclude that whether NH_3 takes part in composing the coordination compound and whether the bond between NH_3 and Cu^{2+} is stable.

The stability of coordination compounds

Estimate the phenomena of following tests based on the involved solubility product constants and stability constants.

Perform the consecutive operations, observe and record the result of each step, then write out the reaction equations.

(1) Put 3—4 drops of 0.1mol/L $AgNO_3$ solution in a tube, then add equal volume of 0.1mol/L NaCl solution.

(2) Add 2 drops of concentrated ammonia solution to solution(a).

(3) Add 2 drops of 0.1mol/L KBr solution to solution(b).

(4) Add 2 drops of 0.5mol/L $Na_2S_2O_3$ solution to 3 solution(c).

(5) Add 2 drops of 0.1mol/L KI solution to solution(d).

(6) Add 2 drops of 0.5mol/L KCN solution to solution(e).

Relation between the formation of complex ion and solution pH

(1) The pH change during: formation of coordination compounds.

Put 2mL of 0.1mol/L $CaCl_2$ solution into one test-tube, and 2mL of 0.1mol/L EDTA-2 Na solution to another tube, add 1 drop of phenolphthalein to the tubes respectively, acidify the solution with 2mol/L ammonia solution to be red. Mix the two portions of solution together, and observe the color change. Write out the reaction equation and answer: at what conditions the formation of coordination compounds will result in the decreasing of the solution pH?

(2) The effect of pH on complexation equilibria.

(a) The coordination between citrate and Fe^{3+}: Add 1mL of 1mol/L sodium citrate solution to 1mL of 0.1mol/L $FeCl_3$ solution, observe and record the color change. Divide the solution into three portions. One portion is used for blank test. Acidify the second portion with 1mol/L HCl solution and basify the third portion with 1mol/L NaOH. Compare the different color of the three portions, [Fe^{3+} is orange, its coordination compound with citrate is bright yellow to yellow-green, $Fe(OH)_3$ is red brown]. Discuss the stability of coordination compound between citrate and Fe^{3+} in acidic and alkaline solution.

(b) The effect of pH formation of $[Fe(NCS)_6]^{3-}$: Add 1mL of 1mol/L KSCN solution to 4—5 drops of 0.1mol/L $FeCl_3$ solution. Divide the solution into two portions. Add several drops of 1mol/L HCl solution to one portion, and several drops of 1mol/L NaOH solution to another. compare the different color in two portions and record. Discuss the stability of $[K(SCN)_6]^{3-}$ in aciaic and alkaline solution.

The activity of coordination compounds

Mix 10 drops of 0.1mol/L $CrCl_3$ solution with 2mL of 0.1mol/L EDTA-2Na solution, observe whether the color of solution will change and conclude whether there is coordination compound formed (the EDTA complex ion of Cr^{3+} is dark purple). Boil the solution for a few minutes to see whether there is coordination compound formed. Add 1—2 drops of 2mol/L ammonia solution to see whether there are green $Cr(OH)_3$ precipitated. Does the difficulty of forming the EDTA complex ion of Cr^{3+} result from its low stability?

The effect of coordination on redox property

(1) Add 30% H_2O_2 solution to 4—5 drops of $CoCl_2$ solution, observe and record the phenomenon. Can H_2O_2 solution oxide Co^{2+} to brown Co^{3+}?

(2) Add excess concentrated ammonia solution to 4—5 drop of $CoCl_2$ solution until the precipitate dissolves. Observe the. color change. Add H_2O_2 solution to see whether

the color will change. Acidify the solution with 6mol/L HCl solution, observe and record the color change. Explain the effect of formation of complex ion on the reductive property of Co^{2+}.

(3) Put 1mL of $CoCl_2$ solution and 5 drops of starch solution in a test tube, then add iodine solution drop by drop, observe and record the color change. Put 2 drops of $CoCl_2$ solution in another test tube, add excess KCN solution until the formed precipitate dissolves, then add 5 drops of starch solution and add iodine solution drop by drop, observe and record the color change. Write out the reaction equations and discuss the effect of KCN on reductive property of Co^{2+}.

Masking

Masking Fe^{3+} with F^-: Into a tube containing a few drops of 0.1mol/L $FeCl_3$ solution, add several drops of 1mol/L KSCN solution, then add solid NaF, shake the tube to dissolve NaF. Record the color of the solution and write out the reaction equation.

Into another tube containing a few drops of 0.5mol/L $CoCl_2$ solution, add several drops of KSCN solution, then add equal volume of acetone, blue $[Co(SCN)_4]^{2-}$ is formed which indicates the presence of Co^{2+}. Add solid NaF to the blue solution and observe whether the blue color will disappear.

Design a test to detect Co^{2+} in the presence of Fe^{3+}.

Formation of chelate

Forming a chelate of $[Cu(P_2O_7)_2]^{6-}$: Add $K_4P_2O_7$ solution dropwise to two drops of 0.1mol/L $CuSO_4$ solution until the precipitate dissolve to produce a dark blue solution.

$$2Cu^{2+} + P_2O_7^{4-} = Cu_2P_2O_7 \downarrow$$
$$Cu_2P_2O_7 + 3P_2O_7^{4-} = 2[Cu(P_2O_7)_2]^{6-}$$

The structure of $[Cu(P_2O_7)_2]^{6-}$ is showed below:

```
           O              O         6-
           ‖              ‖
       O—P=O          O—P=O
           |        ↘    |
           O       Cu    O
           |      ↗      |
       O=P—O          O=P—O
           ‖              ‖
           O              O
```

Instructions

Requirements

(1) What are complex ions and coordination compounds?

(2) What set of conditions should be needed to produce coordination compounds?

(3) How to prove that $[Cu(NH_3)_4]^{2+}$ is formed in the experiment?

(4) Show the differences between coordination compounds and double salts with laboratory methods.

(5) What properties of the substance will change when coordination compounds are formed

(6) Explain the intrinsic property of the bonds in coordination compounds.

(7) How to judge the relative stability of various coordination compounds?

(8) What factors will influence the stability of coordination compounds?

(9) Compare the similarity and differences between chelant and complexant.

(10) Add KSCN solution to ferric solution prior to the addition of EDTA solution, explain what will happen to the mixture.

Notes

(1) Special care should be taken with the highly poisonous KSCN, and the solution should be recollected after the experiment.

(2) During the-preparation of $[Cu(NH_3)_4]SO_4$, ammonia solution should be added to the solution only when the solid $CuSO_4$ dissolved completely. And the ammonia solution should be concentrated.

Report format

(1) Objectives.

(2) Procedure.

(a) Show the contents with-reaction equations and flow charts.

(b) Give concise conclusions to each test.

Questions

(1) Does the complexation equilibria is same to other chemical equilibria?

(2) Show the sameness between the complexation equilibrium of coordination compound and the dissolve equilibrium of precipitate.

(3) Does there exist common ion effect in the complexation equilibrium?

(4) Which elements are prone to form coordination compounds?

Yao Jun

EXPERIMENT FOURTEEN

The Properties of Halogen

Objectives

1. Master the methods of how to prepare halogens and the general principles.

2. Learn how to identify the halogen ions.

3. Validate (test) the physical and chemical properties of halogens, haloid oxyacid, haloid oxysalt and hydrogen halide.

Principles

1. Group Ⅶ elements comprise of fluorine F, chlorine Cl, bromine Br, iodine I and astatine $_{85}$At, which have similar structure of the outer and penultimate electron layers. The presence of one unpaired electron determines its likeness to get one electron, forming corresponding halogenide. All halogens have active nonmetallic characters with a usual oxidation state of ion -1, but the oxidation states in the haloid oxyacid are displayed as $+1$, $+3$, $+5$, $+7$.

2. Free halogen molecule (such as Cl_2, Br_2, I_2) each is obtained by oxidizing its corresponding halogenide.

3. All the halogen molecules are oxidants with different chemical activity according to the sequence as $F_2 > Cl_2 > Br_2 > I_2$. Whereas all halogen ions are reducers with their reducing activity decreasing in the following series: $I^- > Br^- > Cl^- > F^-$.

4. Halogen molecules are non-polar so that they are readily soluble in some non-polar solvents (organic solvents). Especially iodine is soluble in KI solution due to the form of $KI \cdot I_2$ molecules.

5. Most ionic halogenides are readily soluble in water except silver halide (AgX), which is also insoluble in dilute nitric acid (HNO_3) solution. But compounds of Ag^+ with CO_3^{2-}, PO_4^{3-}, CrO_4^{2-} all readily dissolve in HNO_3 solution. So silver halide (AgX) can be precipitated in HNO_3, solution as to prevent the disturbance from the other anions.

6. Diverseness of the solubility of AgX in ammonia solution ($NH_3 \cdot H_2O$) determines the density of NH_3 is useful to separate the mixed haloid ions. For example, $(NH_3)_2CO_3$ is added to dissolve AgCl, and separated from AgBr and AgI. The relative reaction equations are given below:

$$(NH_3)_2CO_3 + H_2O \longrightarrow NH_4HCO_3 + NH_3H_2O$$
$$AgCl + 2NH_3 \cdot H_2O \longrightarrow [Ag(NH_3)_2]^+ + Cl^- + 2H_2O$$

7. All the haloid oxyacid radicals have oxidizing activity. Among them hypochlorous acid (HClO) is the strongest oxidant. It is usually used as bleacher and antiseptic because of its capacity of bleaching and sterilizing.

Equipment

Centrifugal tube, centrifugal machine.

Chemicals

Solid: $I_2(s)$, red phosphor, zinc powder, KCl, KBr, KI, MnO_2, $KClO_3$.

Acid: H_2SO_3 3mol/L, 18mol/L; HCl 12mol/L, HNO_3 6mol/L.

Salt: KBr 0.1mol/L; KClO. 1mol/L; KI 0.1mol/L; $AgNO_3$ 0.1mol/L; NaClO solution; I_2 solution; Chloroform ($CHCl_3$)

Test paper: Blue litmus test paper, $Pb(Ac)_2$ test paper, filter paper, KI / amylum test paper

Iodine reaction with metallic and nonmetallic elements

1. Iodine solution reaction with zinc powder. Add a spoon of zinc powder to a test tube containing 1mL of iodine solution. Shake sufficiently (in contrast to another test tube with only 1mL of iodine solution). Observe the color change of iodine solution (heated if the phenomenon is not obvious). Write out the chemical reaction equations and explain the result above.

2. Iodine reaction with red phosphor (P). Mix some $I_2(s)$ with red P into a test paper, and then add 1—2 drops of water (when I_2 is dry). Strong reaction may occurs after the test tube is heated in water bath. Then put a piece of wet litmus paper near the top of the tube to detect the product (HI). Record the phenomenon, write out the chemical reaction equations and explain the result above.

Comparing the oxidizing activity of Cl_2, Br_2 and I_2

1. Comparing the oxidizing activity of Cl_2 and I_2. Add a drop of 0.1mol/L KI solution to a test tube, and then dilute it with about 1mL of distilled water. Continuously add aqueous solution of chlorine drop by drop, observe the color change. Then add 1mL

chloroform ($CHCl_3$), shake, and observe the color of $CHCl_3$ layer. Go on to add superfluous aqueous solution of chlorine until the color of $CHCl_3$ layer disappears. Write out the chemical reaction equations and explain the result above.

2. Comparing the oxidizing activity of Br_2 and I_2. Add drops of aqueous solution of bromine to a test tube containing 1mL 0.1mol/L KBr solution, and then add drops of amylum solution. Record the phenomenon and write out the chemical reaction equation and explain the result above.

3. Comparing the oxidizing activity of Cl_2 and Br_2. Add drops of aqueous solution of chlorine to a test tube containing 1mL 0.1mol/L KBr solution; observe the color change of the solution. Then add 1mL $CHCl_3$ while shaking, observe the color of the $CHCl_3$ layer again. Write out the chemical reaction equations and explain the result above.

Summarize the experimental results above, then range the halogen molecules (Cl_2, Br_2, I_2) conforming to their oxidizing activity whether increasing or decreasing. Illustrate that rule with standard electrode potentials.

Preparation of the halogens

Add some KCl, KBr and KI crystals to three dry tubes respectively, then add 2mL 3mol/L H_2SO_4 and some MnO_2 to each tube. Put a piece of KI/ amylum paper near the top of the tube containing KCl to detect the emitted gas (Cl_2). Finally add 1mL $CHCl_3$ to the other two tubes and observe the color of $CHCl_3$ layer carefully. Write out the chemical reaction equations and explain the result above.

Comparing the reducing activity of the hydrogen halogen

1. Add a few KCl particles to a dry test tube, then 2—3 drops of concentrated sulfuric acid (H_2SO_4) are added. Observe what occurs in the tube, put a piece of blue litmus test paper near the top of tube to detect the emitted gas (HCl).

2. Add a few KBr particles to a dry test tube, and then 2—3 drops of concentrated sulfuric acid (H_2SO_4) are added. Observe what occurs in the tube, put a piece of test paper moistened with solution of I_2 near the top of tube to detect the emitted gas (SO_2).

3. Add a few KI particles to a dry test tube, then 2—3 drops of concentrated sulphuric acid (H_2SO_4) are added. Observe what occurs in the tube, put a piece of blue Pb(Ac)$_2$ test paper near the top of tube to detect the emitted gas (H_2S).

Summarize the three different products above, then range the halide ions (Cl^-, Br^-, I^-) according to their reducing activity while increasing or decreasing. Illustrate that rule with standard electrode potential.

The oxidizing activity of hypochlorites and chlorates

1. Add 1mL of 0.1mol/L KI solution and 1mL of $CHCl_3$, then add 1—2 drops of natrium hypochlorite (NaClO) solution and shake sufficiently. Observe the color of the $CHCl_3$ layer. Then add superfluous NaClO solution drop by drop while shaking until the color of the $CHCl_3$ layer disappears. Write out the chemical reaction equations and explain the result above.

2. Add some potassium chlorates ($KClO_3$) crystals into a test tube, and then dissolve them in 1—2mL of water. Continuously add 10 drops of 0.1mol/L KI solution. Then divided into two tubes mixture solution above, one of which is acidified by concentrated H_2SO_4, another is held for comparison. Wait a minute, observe any change between them. Try to conclude the difference of the oxidizing activity of the chlorates in different medium, e.g., in a neutral solution or in an acidic solution.

Instructions

Requirements

(1) Why are the oxidation states of the halogens in their singulars compounds? Please relate the atom structure to explain it.

(2) Explain why the oxidizing activity is decreasing as follows: $F_2 > Cl_2 > Br_2 > I_2$, but the reducing activity is increasing as follows: $F^- < Cl^- < Br^- < I^-$.

(3) Which reaction can be selected to prepare a small quantity of Cl_2, Br_2, I_2 in the lab?

(4) Enumerate the main chemical properties of the free halogen molecules.

(5) What rules do the reducing activity of the hydrogen halogenides obey? How to detect HCl (g), SO_2 and H_2S?

Operation

(1) Separate the precipitate by centrifuge.

(2) Examine whether the precipitate is completely subsided.

(3) Detect the small quantity of the emitted gas from the test tube.

(4) Extract a small quantity of liquid in the test tube.

Report format

(1) Objectives.

(2) Procedures (Table 13).

Table 13　Procedures

sample	chemicals	phenomenon	reaction equation

conclusion			

Questions

(1) Illuminate the difference of oxidizing activity of oxychlorates with the different oxidation states of chlorine. What do you think of "Increasing oxidation state means increasing oxidizing activity"?

(2) How to detect the solution containing I^-?

Sun Lian

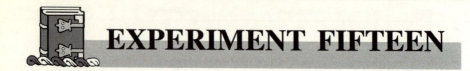

EXPERIMENT FIFTEEN

Preparation of Medicinal Sodium Chloride and Examination of Impurities Limitation

Objectives

1. To master principle and method of how to prepare medicinal sodium chloride.
2. To learn how to identify and check medicines.

Principles

1. Sodium chloride is soluble in aqueous solution, so the impurities in sodium chloride can be removed with the processes showed below:

(1) The insoluble impurities are removed by filtration.

(2) Some soluble impurities can be removed by precipitation basing on their chemical properties. For example, sulfate can be separated as $BaSO_4$ by solution of $BaCl_2$; Ca^{2+}, Mg^{2+}, Ba^{2+}, Fe^{3+} etc. can be removed as insoluble precipitates.

(3) Some low content soluble impurities, such as Br^-, I^-, K^+, having different solubility from sodium chloride, can be removed by recrystallization. They will be retained in the mother liquid and moved away.

2. The limit tests of barium, sulfate, potassium, calcium and magnesium are carried out in comparison tubes by addition of corresponding precipitate agents. Under same conditions, any opalescence produced in the test solutions should not be pronounced than that of the reference solutions.

3. Heavy metals (comprising the ions of Pb, Bi, Cu, Hg, Sb, Sn, Co, Zn and other metals) can be colored by sulfide ion under the specified test conditions. The test of heavy metallic impurities is carried out by comparing the color of solutions with the corresponding reference solution under same conditions.

Equipment

Electric cooker, evaporating dish, Buchner funnel, platinum wire, beakers (250mL), platform balance, color-comparison tubes (25mL, 50mL).

Chemicals

Solid: raw sodium chloride

Acid: concentrated hydrochloric acid, dilute hydrochloric acid (1/50mol/L), sulfuric acid(6mol/L)

Alkali: sodium hydroxide solution (2mol/L, 1/50mol/L), saturated solution of sodium carbonate.

Salt: $BaCl_2$(25%), KI(10%), Ca^{2+} TS, $AgNO_3$(0.25mol/L), KBr(10%), Mg^{2+} TS, zinc uranylacetate solution, $(NH_4)_2C_2O_4$ TS, Na_2HPO_4 TS, NH_4Cl TS, ammonia TS

Others: KT-starch test paper, bromothymol blue TS

Procedures

Purification of NaCl

The procedure is illustrated as the following flow chart.

Raw NaCl (impurities: organic compounds, sludge, sand, Ca^{2+}, Mg^{2+}, Fe^{3+}, SO_4^{2-}, Br^-, I^-, etc.)

↓ heat moderately to carbonize the organic impurities
↓ dissolve the solid is a beaker while warming
↓ filter with suction by tilt-pour process ↓ while hot

filter residue (sludge, sand, carbonaceous deposit)

filtrate
↓ heat to keep the solution on the simmer
↓ add 25% $BaCl_2$ solution drop by drop on stirring
↓ boil and cool down, filter by tilt-pour process

filter residue reject ($BaSO_4$)

filtrate
↓ heat
↓ add saturated solution of Na_2CO_3, then add solution of NaOH to adjust the pH to 10—11
↓ boil, and cool down, filter by tilt-pour process

mother liquid (saturated solution of NaCl containing Br^-, I^-, K^+)

filtrate
↓ neutralize with HCl until the pH 3—4
↓ Vapor the solution to be thick paste, a lot of crystal precipitate
↓ vacuum filter while hot

Figure 1   Raw NaCl

```
                              ↓ vacuum filter while hot
──────────────────────────────────────────────────────
    filter residue                    crude NaCl
    reject (CaCO₃, BaCO₃,             ↓ recrystallize refined NaCl
    Fe(OH)₃, Mg(OH)₂, 3MgCO₃)         ↓ dry
                           ────────────────
                    mother liquid (recycled)    product
```

Continute figure 1   Raw NaCl

Identification test

An aqueous solution (1 in 20) of the product is prepared for the identification test.

1. Sodium.

(1) Dry test (flame color): prepare a platinum wire by burning it on a non-luminous flame after moistening it with concentrated hydrochloric acid until the flame is colorless. Moisten the test solution on the platinum wire; it imparts an intense yellow color to a non-luminous flame.

(2) Precipitation: add 2 drops of solution in a tube, acidified with three drops of 3mol/L acetic acid, and add 10 drops of zinc uranylacetate TS, if necessary, rub the inside wall of the test tube with a glass rod. A yellow precipitate is formed.

$$Na^+ + Zn^{2+} + 3UO_2^{2+} + 8Ac^- + HAc + 9H_2O \rightarrow Zn(Ac)_2 \cdot 3UO_2 \cdot 9H_2O + H^+$$

2. Chloride. 2 drops of the tested solution yield a white, curdy precipitate with 2 drops of 0.25mol/L silver nitrate TS. On addition of 6mol/L ammonia TS, the precipitate dissolve. White precipitate is formed again by acidifing the solution with 6mol/L nitric acid:

$$Cl^- + Ag^+ \rightarrow AgCl \downarrow$$
$$AgCl \downarrow + 2NH_3 \rightarrow Ag(NH_3)_2^+ + Cl^-$$
$$Ag(NH_3)_2^+ + Cl^- + 2H^+ \rightarrow AgCl \downarrow + 2NH_4^+$$

Limit test of impurity

The product should be checked with the limit tests described below.

(1) Appearance of solution: dissolve 5g in 25mL of distilled water. The solution should be clear and colorless.

(2) Acidity or alkalinity: dissolve 5g in carbon dioxide-free water, and mute with the same solvent to 50mL. Add 2 drops of bromothymol blue TS: Not more than 0.1mL of 0.02mol/L hydrochloric acid (HCl) or 0.02mol/L sodium hydroxide (NaOH) is required to change the color of the solution.

The content of free acid or alkali, if there is any, in medicinal NaCl should not be more than the limit. And the pH range of bromothymol blue is 6.0—7.6, yellow to blue.

(3) Iodide(I^-) and bromide(Br^-): dissolve 1g in 3mL of distilled water and add 1mL of chloroform. Cautiously introduce, dropwise, with constant agitation, dilute chlorine(Cl_2) TS(1 in 2): the chloroform does not acquire a violet, yellow, or orange color.

Control test: add 1mL of 10% iodide TS and bromide TS in two tubes respectively, the following step is similar to that of the test solution. The color of chloroform in one tube, (containing the iodide TS) is violet while the other tube is yellow or orange.

$$2Br^- + Cl_2 \rightarrow Br_2 + 2Cl^-$$
$$2I^- + Cl_2 \rightarrow I_2 + 2Cl^-$$

(4) Barium(Ba^{2+}): dissolve 4.0g in 20mL of distilled water, filter if necessary, and divide the solution into two equal portion. To one portion add 2mL of diluted sulfuric acid, and to the other add 2mL of water the solution should be equally clear after standing for 2 hours.

(5) Calcium(Ca^{2+}) and magnesium(Mg^{2+}): dissolve 4g in 20mL of distilled water, add 2mL of ammonia TS and divide the mixture into two equal portions. Treat one portion with 1ml of ammonium oxalate TS and the other portion with 1mL of dibasic sodium phosphate TS and a few drops of ammonium chloride TS: no opalescence is produced within 5minutes.

Control test: calcium-Pipet 1mL of calcium TS to a tube, alkalied with ammonia TS, add ammonium oxalate TS: while crystal is precipitated.

$$Ca^{2+} + C_2O_4^{2-} \rightarrow CaC_2O_4 \downarrow$$

Magnesium-Pipet 1mL of magnesium TS to a tube, add a few drops of ammonia TS and ammonium chloride, drop in dibasic sodium phosphate (Na_2HPO_4) TS: white precipitate is separated from the solution.

$$Mg^{2+} + HPO_4^{2-} + NH_4^+ + OH^- \rightarrow MgNH_4PO_4 \downarrow + H_2O$$

(6) Sulfate (SO_4^{2-}): reference preparation into a 50mL color-comparison tube pipet 1mL of standard potassium sulfate solution, and dilute with water to about 35mL. Add 5mL of 1mol/L hydrochloric acid and 5mL of barium chloride TS. Dilute with water to volume and mix.

Test preparation into 50mL, color-comparison tube place 5g of the product, and dissolve the solid with about 35mL of distilled water, filter if necessary. Add 5mL of barium chloride TS, dilute with water to volume and mix.

Procedure-allow the two tubes to stand for 10minutes, and view downward. Any opalescence produced in the latter tube is -not more pronounced than that of the standard tube.

Standard potassium sulfate dissolve 0.1813g of potassium chloride with distilled water in 1000mL volumetric flask, dilute with water to volume and mix. This solution contains the equivalent of 0.1mg of sulfate per mL.

(7) Iron: dissolve 5g with 35mL of distilled water in & 50mL color-comparison tube, add 5mL of dilute hydrochloric acid and approximate 30mg of ammonium persulfate, add 3mL of 30% ammonium thiocyanate (NH_4SCN) solution and sufficient water to produce 50mL, mix well. Any color produced is not more intense than that of a reference solution using 1.5mL of standard iron solution (0.0003%).

$$Fe^{3+} + 3SCN^- \rightarrow Fe(SCN)_3$$

Standard iron solution-dissolve 863.0mg of ferric ammonium sulfate in water, add 2mL of dilute hydrochloric acid, and dilute with water to 1000ml pipet 10mL of this solution into a 100mL volumetric flask, add 0.5mL of dilute hydrochloric acid, dilute with water to volume, and mix. This solution contains the equivalent of 0.01mg of iron per mL.

(8) Potassium (K^+): dissolve 5g of product with distilled water in a color-comparison tube, and adjust with 2 drops of acetic acid to a pH between 5 and 6. Add 2mL of 0.1mol/L sodium tetraphenylboron solution and dilute with water to 50mL, mix. Any opalescence produced is not more pronounced than that of a reference solution using 0.5mL of standard potassium sulfate solution (0.02%).

$$K^+ + B(C_6H_5)_4^- \rightarrow KB(C_6H_5)_4 \downarrow$$

Standard potassium sulfate solution Dissolve 2.2280g of potassium sulfate, previously dried at 105℃ and weighed accurately, with water in 1000mL volumetric flask, dilute to volume, and mix. This solution contains the equivalent of 1mg of potassium per mL.

Sodium tetraphenylboron solution Triturate 1.5g of sodium tetraphenylboron with 10mL of water, then add 40mL of water triturate again and filter.

(9) Heavy metals: reference preparation into a 50mL color-comparison tube pipet 1mL of standard lead solution (20μg of Pb), add 2mL of-dilute acetic acid and dilute with water to 25mL.

Test preparation dissolve 5g of the product with 23mL of distilled water in another 50mL add 2mL of dilute acetic acid.

Procedure To each of the two tubes add 10mL of hydrogen sulfide TS, dilute to 50mL and mix. The tubes are allowed to stand for 10minutes in dark place. If the color of the solution from the standard preparation is not darker than that of the solution from the standard preparation, it pronounces that the content of heavy metals is not more than the limits.

Instructions

Requirements

(1) What impurities are contained in raw solid of sodium chloride? And how to remove these. impurities?

(2) Why, during the purification of NaCl, should the agents be added sequentially: $BaCl_2$, Na_2CO_3, and HCl? Can we change the order of agents?

(3) How to remove the impurities of K^+, Br^-, I^- and otter ions?

(4) To remove SO_4^{2-}, Ca^{2+}, Mg^{2+} etc as precipitate by addition corresponding precipitate agents, what influence does heating or not heating the solution have on the result? How to determine whether these ions are removed entirely?

(5) How to remove the excess precipitate ages: $BaCl_2$, Na_2CO_3 and NaOH?

(6) During they adjustment of pH of the solution with HCl, what can we deal with the excess HCl? Why should we adjust the solution to be weak acidic? Can we adjust the solution to be weak alkaline?

(7) Can we evaporate the condensed solution to dryness? Why?

(8) What is recrystallization? How much water should be appropriate to dissolve the product during recrystallization?

(9) Can tap water be used to dissolve the resulting product we check the impurity limitation? Why?

Operation

(1) Precipitate impurity ions and check whether the ions precipitate completely

(2) Vacuum filter(filter with suction)

(3) Evaporate solution and crystallize

(4) Recrystallize

Notes

(1) Water used to dissolve the material should be proportioned to the material. Too much water will introduce difficult to the following : evaporation.

(2) When we remove the impurities by addition precipitate agents, the time of boiling should not be too long. Otherwise, some of NaCl will separate from the hot solution. If some NaCl crystal, some few distilled water should be added to the solution.

(3) During evaporation, the crystal membrane of NaCl on the surface of the condensed solution should be ruptured with a parallel lying glass rod, otherwise, the crystal will splatter everywhere.

(4) Some soluble impurities, such as: Br^-, I^- and K^+, will be removed away together with the mother liquid. So the solution should not be evaporated to dryness. Furthermore, the resulting crystal shad be pressed with a glass stopper during filtration.

(5) Use the comparison tubes correctly. And compare the sample tubes with the corresponding standard tubes under same conditions.

Report format

(1) Objectives.

(2) Principle.

(3) Procedure (illustrated with a flow chart).

(4) The yield of refined NaCl and its percentage yield.

(5) Write out the reaction equations of identification of Na^+, Cl^-. And illustrate the results of impurity limit tests with a table.

Questions

Summarize the results of the tests and give conclusion on how to get a higher yield.

Li Gairu

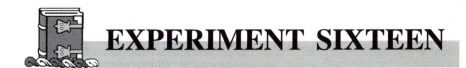

EXPERIMENT SIXTEEN

Preparation of Ferrous Ammonium Sulfate Hexahydrate (FAS)

Objectives

1. To master the operation of heating in the water bath and filter by suction.
2. To learn how to prepare double salts.

Principle

The ferrous ion is converted into ferric ion easily when it is open to the air, but the ferrous ion in FAS cannot be easily oxidized.

Ferrous sulfate ($FeSO_4$), which can be obtained by reacting iron powder with diluted sulfuric acid (H_2SO_4), reacts with ammonium sulfate (($NH_4)_2SO_4$) in equimolar ratio in aqueous solution. Ferrous ammonium sulfate hexahydrate ($FeSO_4 \cdot (NH_4)_2SO_4 \cdot 6H_2O$), with less solubility, crystallizes from the solution as pale blue monoclinic crystal.

$$Fe + H_2SO_4 = FeSO_4 + H_2 \uparrow$$
$$FeSO_4 + (NH_4)_2SO_4 + 6H_2O = FeSO_4 \cdot (NH_4)_2SO_4 \cdot 6H_2O$$

Equipment

Platform balance, graduated cylinder (10mL), Erlenmeyer flask, filter flask, Buchner funnel, evaporating dish, thermostatic water bath, comparison tube (25mL).

Chemicals

Iron powder, ammonia sulfate [$(NH_4)_2SO_4$]; H_2SO_4 3mol/L; HCl 3mol/L, 10% Na_2CO_3 Solution; KSCN 0.1mol/L solution.

Procedures

Procedures

(1) Place 2g iron powder and 20mL 10% Na_2CO_3 into an Erlenmeyer flask, and

heated over an electric cooker for about 10 minutes. Remove the solution by tilt-pour process; wash the iron powder with distiller water.

(2) Add 15mL 3mol/L H_2SO_4 into the Erlenmeyer flask, heat in the water bath at 60—70℃ until the reaction is completed. Filter by suction while hot; wash the residue with 5mL of warm water. The filtrate is put into a clean evaporating dish. On the basis of the remaining iron powder, calculate the ferrous sulfate's theoretical yield.

(3) For 0.1g of ferric sulfate, 0.075g ammonia sulfate was added as solid reagent into an evaporating dish. Stir the mixture to dissolve the ammonia sulfate. Then heat the evaporating dish in the boiling water bath until a layer of tiny crystals is observed. Cool the solution and filter by suction. Dry the pale blue crystals and weigh it. Calculate the percentage yield of the product.

Purity examination of the product

Dissolve 2g of ferrous ammonium sulfate hexahydrate with 30mL of oxygen-free distilled water in a 50mL flask for comparison. Add 4mL of 3mol/L HCl and 2mL of 0.1mol/L KSCN. Fill to the mark with oxygen-free distilled water and mix the solution. Compare the color with that of a series of standard samples to determine the purity grade of the product.

Preparation of the standard sample

Add 30mL solution containing ferric ion (the content of Fe^{3+} in various solutions are shown below) into comparison tubes. The following procedure is same as that for the product.

Grade I : 0.10mg.
Grade II : 0.20mg.
Grade III : 0.30mg.

Instructions

Requirements

(1) How to get rid of the oil from the iron powder?

(2) How to determine whether the reaction to produce ferric sulfate is completed?

(3) The solution of ferrous sulfate is easy to be oxidized. How to prevent the oxidation for preparing the ferrous ammonium sulfate hexahydrate?

(4) How to calculate the yield of the product?

(5) How to get oxygen-free distilled water? Why should the oxygen-free distilled water being used to dissolve the ferrous ammonium sulfate hexahydrate?

Operation

(1) Master the operation of filtration by suction.

(2) Practice washing solid by tilt-pour process.

(3) Understand the analytical method of impurity limitation.

Report format

(1) Objectives.

(2) Principle.

(3) Procedures:

(a) Illustrate the procedure with a flow chart.

(b) Calculate the theoretic yield of $FeSO_4 \cdot 7H_2O$ and FAS.

(c) Percentage yield.

(d) Purity examination.

Notes

(1) After ammonium sulfate was added to the evaporating dish, the mixture must be stirred thoroughly until the ammonium sulfate dissolves.

(2) The time for evaporation should not be too long and the concentrate should be kept under room temperature for a while to produce the crystal of $FeSO_4 \cdot (NH_4)_2SO_4 \cdot 6H_2O$.

Questions

(1) Which should be present in considerable excess between the iron powder and the sulfuric acid in the secondary step?

(2) Why the solution should be filtered while it is still hot, when the reaction for ferric sulfate is complete? Why do we need warm water to wash the filter residue?

(3) Why should the pH of the solution be kept at 2 or 3 during evaporation?

Sun Lian

EXPERIMENT SEVENTEEN

Preparation and Content Assay of Zinc Gluconate

Objectives

1. To learn how to prepare Zinc gluconate.
2. To learn bow to determine the concentration of zinc salt.

Principles

Calcium gluconate reacts with equal molar of zinc sulfate:

$$Ca(C_6H_{11}O_7)_2 + ZnSO_4 \longrightarrow Zn(C_6H_{11}O_7)_2 + CaSO_4$$

Equipment

Platform balance, measuring cylinder, beaker, evaporating dish, electric cooker, acid-type buret, thermostatic water bath.

Chemicals

Calcium gluconate, heptahydrate zinc sulfate, 95% ethanol, ammonia-ammonium chloride buffer solution, 0.1mol/L disodium ethylenediaminetetraacetate standard solution, eriochrome black solution.

Procedures

Preparation procedure of Zinc gluconate

Measure 80mL water to a beaker, heat it to 80—90℃, then add 13.4g of eriochrume black solution, $ZnSO_4 \cdot 7H_2O$ and allow them to be dissolved completely. Put the beaker in water bath and keep heating at 90℃, add 20g of calcium gluconate gradually and then mix constantly. After 30 minutes, filter it quickly by vacuum filter (double filter paper). The filtrate was transferred to an evaporating dish (filter cake discarded). and concentrated to approximately 20mL. Then the filtrate is cooled to room temperature. 20mL of 95% ethanol is added to reduce the solubility of zinc gluconate and it is stirred continually. A lot of colloidal zinc gluconate was separated out. After stirring completely, the precipitate changed slowly into crystal then by filtering. The crude product is obtained on filtration. It is dissolved by adding 20mL water at 90℃, filter warmly, then cool the filtrate to room temperature. Add 20mL of 95% ethanol, stir strongly, and the crystal was separated out. After filtering and baking the crystals at 50℃, pure product was obtained.

Content assay

Dissolve 0.8g of zinc gluconate, accurately weighed, in 20mL of water (sometimes need to be heated). Add 10mL of ammonia-ammonium chloride buffer solution and 4 drops of eriochrome black solution and titrate with 0.1mol/L disodium ethylenediaminetetraacetate (EDTA) standard solution, until the solution is deep blue in color. The zinc concentration in the sample can be calculated as follows:

$$Zn\% = \frac{C_{EDTA} \times V_{EDTA} \times 65}{W \times 1000} \times 100\%$$

$(CV)_{EDTA}$ is the concentration of EDTA (C, mol/L) and volume (V, mL); W_S is the weight of the sample (g).

Instructions

Requirements

(1) Design flow chart of the preparation of zinc gluconate.

(2) Why must we keep the temperature at 90℃ when zinc sulfate reacts with calcium gluconate?

(3) By how many means can zinc gluconate be recrystallized?

(4) How can zinc content of zinc gluconate be determined?

Operation

(1) Master the operation of thermostatic water bath.

(2) Learn the recrystallization method with ethanol as a solvent.

Report format

(1) Objectives.

(2) Principles (in reaction formula).

(3) Flow chart of preparation.

(4) Yield, percentage yield.

(5) Record data and result dealing.

		1	2
record part	$W_{(zinc\ gluconate)}/g$		
	$C_{EDTA}/(mol \cdot L^{-1})$		
	V_{EDTA}/mL		
	Molar weight of zinc/$(g \cdot mol^{-1})$		
calculation	$Zn\% = \dfrac{C_{EDTA} \times V_{EDTA} \times 65}{W \times 1000} \times 100\%$		

Notes

(1) The reaction must be undertaken at constant temperature water bath of 90℃. Higher temperature may lead to the decomposition of zinc gluconate while too low temperature may cause the reduction of the solubility of zinc gluconate.

(2) When recrystallized with ethanol as solvent, any amount of zinc gluconate may appear at the beginning. Chopstick, easy to stir, often replaces glass rod.

(3) The filtrate is concentrated in boiled water bath.

(4) When titrating with 0.1mol/L disodium EDTA standard solution, observe color change carefully.

Questions

(1) Design flow chart for the preparation of zinc gluconate.

(2) Why must we keep the temperature at 90℃ when zinc sulfate reacts with calcium gluconate?

Chang Junmin

EXPERIMENT EIGHTEEN

Synthesis of Copper Sulfate Pentahydrate

Objectives

1. To learn the principles and procedures for the synthesis of copper sulfate pentahydrate using copper waste and industrial sulfuric acid.

2. To further enhance the basic inorganic synthesis skills such as combustion, heating with water bath, vacuum filtration and crystallization.

Principles

$CuSO_4 \cdot 5H_2O$ is readily soluble in water and insoluble in absolute alcohol. It dehydrates when heated.

There are many methods to synthesize $CuSO_4 \cdot 5H_2O$, including electrolysis and oxidation. In this experiment, copper waste and industrial sulfuric acid are used as starting materials to synthesize $CuSO_4 \cdot 5H_2O$. Copper powder is first combusted to form copper oxide, and then copper oxide is dissolved in sulfuric acid of proper concentration. The chemical equations are as follows:

$$2Cu + O_2 \xrightarrow{combustion} 2CuO(black)$$
$$CuO + H_2SO_4 \longrightarrow CuSO_4 + H_2O$$

There are a number of other soluble and insoluble impurities formed in the reaction solution, due to the impurities in copper waste and industrial sulfuric acid in addition to the formation of copper sulfate. The insoluble impurities can be removed by filtration. Typically oxidizing agents (such as H_2O_2) are first used to oxidize Fe^{2+} to Fe^{3+} to remove soluble impurities. Then the pH value is adjusted to 3. The pH of solution should not be more than 4, otherwise, alkaline copper sulfate may precipitate out. After the solution is heated to boil, Fe^{3+} hydrolyzes to form $Fe(OH)_3$ precipitate and then it is removed. The chemical equations are as follows:

$$2Fe^{2+} + 2H^+ + H_2O_2 \longrightarrow 2Fe^{3+} + 2H_2O$$
$$Fe^{3+} + 3H_2O \longrightarrow Fe(OH)_3 \downarrow + 3H^+$$

The purified $CuSO_4$ solution is evaporated, cooled to crystallize and vacuum filtered to obtain blue $CuSO_4 \cdot 5H_2O$.

Equipment

Weighing balance, Bunsen burner, porcelain crucible, crucible tongs, triangle, Buchner funnel, filter flask, beaker, TLC plates, glass rod, graduated cylinder, evaporation dish, filter paper and scissors.

Chemicals

Copper powder, H_2SO_4 (3mol/L), H_2O_2 (3%), $K_3[Fe(CN)_6]$ (0.1mol/L), $CuCO_3$ (C.P), pH litmus paper.

Procedures

Synthesis of copper oxide

The porcelain crucible is cleaned, thoroughly dried by combustion and then cooled to room temperature. 3.0g of copper powder is weighed and placed in the crucible. The crucible is placed on the triangle, mildly and evenly heated with the Bunsen burner. When the Cu powder is dry, the flame is raised to combustion and the crucible is continually stirred. During stirring, the crucible must be held with the tongs to prevent it from falling off the triangle. After the Cu powder is completely converted to black CuO by combustion, stop heating and allow to cool to room temperature.

Preparation of crude $CuSO_4$ solution

The cooled CuO is transferred into a 100mL beaker and mixed with 18mL of 3mol/L H_2SO_4 (industrial purity). The mixture is heated mildly to dissolve the powder.

Purification of $CuSO_4$ solution

Add 2mL of 3% H_2O_2 in dropwise into the crude $CuSO_4$ solution. The mixture is heated and detected for any Fe^{2+} present (how to detect?). After Fe^{2+} is completely oxidized, $CuCO_3$ powder is added slowly and the solution is continually stirred up to pH=3. During this process, the pH of the solution needs to be frequently tested and controlled at pH3, and then the mixture is heated to boil (why?) and filtered while hot under vacuum. The filtrate is transferred into a clean beaker.

Preparation of $CuSO_4 \cdot 5H_2O$ crystals

3mol/L H_2SO_4 is added drop wise to the purified $CuSO_4$ solution to adjust the solation to pH=1. The mixture is transferred to the clean evaporation dish and heated in the water bath until crystal membrane appears on the liquid surface. The mixture is cooled to room temperature and crystallization occurs. The crystals are collected by vacuum filtration and dried with filter paper. Then it is weighed and the yield is calculated.

Questions

1. Why is it necessary to oxidize Fe^{2+} impurities to Fe^{3+} before it is removed from the crude $CuSO_4$ solution? Why does the pH of the solution need to be adjusted to 3? What kind of effect will it have if the pH is too high or too low?

2. Why is it necessary to adjust the pH of purified $CuSO_4$ solution to 1, which is highly acidic?

3. During the evaporation and crystallization of $CuSO_4 \cdot 5H_2O$. Why is necessary to stop heating as soon as the crystal membrane starts to appear until dryness?

4. How to remove residual Cu and CuO from the crucible?

Hai Liqian

EXPERIMENT NINETEEN

Preparation of SnI$_4$

Objectives

1. To learn the inorganic preparation of tin tetraiodide using a non-aqueous solvent (petroleum ethers).
2. To practice basic operations such as refluxing, heating with water bath, etc.

Principles

Tin tetraiodide is a red-orange color, needle-shaped crystal with a density of 4.48g/cm^3, m.p. of 144.5℃, b.p. of 364.5℃ and substantial vapor pressure at 180℃. It is soluble in water and hydrolyzes relatively easily. It decomposes in hot water. It is readily soluble in organic solvents such as carbon disulfide, carbon tetrachloride, benzene and hot petroleum ethers, and its solubility in cold petroleum ethers is relatively low. In solvents such as ethanol, tin tetraiodide reacts with iodides of alkali metals to form black crystalline M$_2$[SnI$_6$] compounds.

Because tin tetraiodide readily hydrolyzes, it is not suitable to be synthesized in aqueous solutions. It is usually dry synthesized, that is, synthesized from the reaction between tin and iodine vapor or with non-aqueous solvents at elevated temperatures. Non-aqueous solvents can be selected from carbon tetrachloride,. glacial acetic acid, etc. In this experiment low-boiling petroleum ethers (b. p. 60—90℃) is used as solvent. It is a mixture of low hydrocarbons (mostly pentanes and hexanes) and is an inert solvent. The synthesis consists of dissolving iodine in petroleum ethers, followed by its reaction with tin metal at elevated temperatures:

$$Sn + 2I_2 = SnI_4$$

Equipment

Weighing balance, round bottom flask (30mL), reflux condenser, beakers (250mL and 30mL), thermometer, constant temperature bath and other heating equipment including ring-stand.

Chemicals

Petroleum ethers (b. p. 60—90℃), tin foil, iodine, 0.1mol/L $AgNO_3$, 0.1mol/L $Pb(NO_3)_2$, saturated KI solution.

Procedures

Preparation of SnI_4

0.5g of crystalline, iodine is weighed with a balance and placed in a clean, dry 30mL round bottom flask. Then 0.2g of tin foils is weighed, cut into small pieces and placed in the same flask followed by the addition of 10mL petroleum ethers. After the reaction apparatus including the reflux condenser is set up, the flask is heated with the water bath until the reaction mixture boils. Temperature of the water bath is controlled to be between 85—95℃, and the flow rate of cooling water is adjusted to keep the condensed liquid to be bellow the middle section of the condenser. Reflux is maintained until the reaction is completed (the color of condensed petroleum ethers solution changes from purple to colorless). The heating is then stopped with the removal of water bath. The condenser is removed when the solution no longer boils. The solution is decanted hot into a clean, dry 30mL beaker, leaving the un-reacted tin foils in-the reaction flask. Residual SnI_4 crystals left on the inside wall of the flask or on the tin foils should be collected with 1—2mL of hot petroleum ethers and then- combined with the solutions in the above-mentioned beaker. The beaker is cooled in an ice bath to start crystallization, When crystallization is complete, the top clear solution (petroleum ethers mother liquor) is carefully decanted into the recycling flask with a glass rod. The small flask containing the crystals is dried with the water bath. The product is weighed and the yield is then calculated.

Property experiments

(1) Small amount of SnI_4 is mixed with 2mL of distilled water. The pH litmus paper is used to test the acidity/causticity of the solution.

(2) The above solution is divided into two test tubes. Several drops of 0.1mol/L $AgNO_3$ is added into one test tube and 0.1mol/L $Pb(NO_3)_2$ into the other test tube. Observe the change and write down the ionic reaction equations.

(3) Small amount of SnI_4 is dissolved with acetone, and the solution is divided into two test tubes. Several drops of water is added into one of the tubes and equal amount of saturated KI solution into the other. Observe and explain.

Questions

1. What effect does it have on the experimental results if the reaction is stopped when the solution boils too violently, condensation is insufficient, iodine and petroleum ethers evaporate from the condenser, or the condensed liquid still has color?

2. Which starting material should be in excess amount in this experiment? Why?

Sun Lian

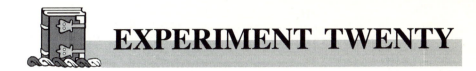

EXPERIMENT TWENTY

Separation and Identification of Methionine and Glycine by Paper Chromatography

Objectives

1. Grasp the basic principle of paper chromatography
2. Grasp the operation of paper chromatography

Principles

Paper chromatography is one of partition chromatography. Filter paper is regarded as the inert carrier. The solid phase is the water absorbed by the paper fiber (about 20% —25%), 6% of which combines with the cellulose's hydroxy into compounds through the H-bonds. Mobile phase is organic solvent. The substances to be separated are distributed between the solid phase and mobile phase. Generally the R_f is used to describe the position of each component in filter paper, as follows:

$$R_f = \frac{\text{distance between the center of the solute zone and the start line}}{\text{distance between the solvent front and the start line}}$$

Under the same experiment condition, the R_f of each component is constant. So the substance can be identified by the R_f value.

In this experiment, the mixture of n-butyl alcohol: ice acetic acid: water (4: 1: 1) is used as mobile phase. Methionine [CH_3—SCH_2—CH_2 CH—(NH_2)—COOH] and glycine [NH_2CH_2COOH] will be developed and separated. The structure of these two compounds is very similar, but the length of the carbon chain for them is different. So their combination ability with water on the filter paper is different. Glycine has stronger polarity than methionine, and moves more slowly on the filter paper. So glycine's R_f is smaller than the methionine's. After development, make them react with ninhydrin under 60℃ and then magenta spots will appear on the paper. The color reaction between a-amino acid and ninhydrin is as follows:

The product's color is blue, purple or magenta.

Equipment

Chromatography tank (or sample tank), middle speed chromatographic paper, capillary (or microsyringe), oven (or electric stove).

Chemicals

Developing solvent: n-butyl alcohol: ice acetic acid: water (4:1:1).
reagent: ninhydrin solution (0.15g ninhydrin + 30mL ice HAc + 50mL acetone).
Methionine standard solution: 0.4mg/mL aqueous solution. Glycine standard solution: 0.4mg/mL aqueous solution. Mixed solution of methionine and glycine.

Procedure

Spotting
Take a middle speed chromatographic paper which is 20cm long and 6cm wide, rile a light starting line 2cm above the bottom in pencil. Draw three " x " on the line and

make the space between "×" 1.5cm. Spot standard solution and sample solution by capillary (or microsyringe) 3—4 times to make the spots' diameter 2mm and air them (or use cold wind to dry them).

Development

Add 35mL developing solvent into the dry chromatographic tank, append the spotted filter paper in the tank and cover it to saturate the paper for 10 minutes. Then dip the paper's edge into the solvent about 0.3—0.5cm and develop it.

Coloration

After the solvent front reaches proper position above starting line (nearly 15cm), take out paper and write down the solvent front by pencil immediately. Allow paper to dry and then spray the ninhydrin solution on it. Put the paper in oven and let coloration last 5min under 60℃, or heat it on the electric stove carefully, and then the magenta spots appear.

Qualitative analysis

Line out the range of spots and find out the center of spots. Measure the distance a between the center and the start line, and the distance b between the start line and the solvent front. Then:

$$R_f = \frac{a}{b}$$

Calculate the R_f of mixture and standard substances respectively, then the components of mixture are identified.

Notes

1. Developing solvent must be prepared in advance and shaken up completely.

2. Each spot must be dry before another spotting and the spot diameter must be 2mm around. Spotting times vary according to the concentration of sample solution.

3. The coloration reagent for amino acid ninhydrin can react with body fluid, for example sweat, so take the edge when pick up the filter paper to avoid impurity in paper.

4. Ninhydrin solution should be prepared before use or stored in refrigerator.

5. The spotted filter paper should not be dipped into the developing solvent during saturation. Carefully dip the paper into the solvent to develop it and avoid the solvent going beyond the starting line.

6. Spray the coloration reagent uniformly and properly to avoid paper being too wet at local site.

Questions

1. What influence the R_f?

2. Why are standard substances often used as reference in the chromatographic experiment?

3. Compare the R_f of the following three acid when the mixed solution of n-butyl alcohol: formic acid: water (10:4:1) was used as developing solvent:

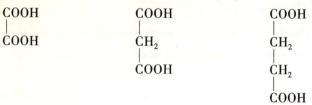

4. How can the paper chromatograms be obtained, which has concentrated spots and orderly solvent front?

5. Why must the filter paper be saturated in chromatography jar before it is dipped into the developing solvent? What is the requirement for time and temperature of saturation?

Sun Lian

EXPERIMENT TWENTY ONE

Synthesis of Potassium Permanganate

Objectives

1. To understand the decomposition of ore by alkali fusion method, and the principles and procedures to synthesize potassium permanganate.
2. To practice basic operations such as extraction, vacuum filtration, evaporation crystallization and recrystallization.
3. To learn to use gas cylinders and reaction apparatus.

Principles

There are multiple methods to synthesize potassium permanganate, and one of them is by using pyrolusite (with MnO_2 as the main component). The synthesis consists of two steps: first, synthesis of potassium manganate by oxidation reactions, followed by conversion of potassium manganate to potassium permanganate. From the electric potential chart, it is known that:

$$E_A^\theta \quad MnO_4^- \text{---} MnO_4^{2-} \text{---} MnO_2$$
$$E_B^\theta \quad MnO_4^- \text{---} MnO_4^{2-} \text{---} MnO_2$$

MnO_4^{2-} is unstable and readily disproportionates in acidic medium. It is less likely to disproportionate in alkaline medium, and the reaction is much slower. Therefore, it is only suitable to be stored in alkaline medium. Alkaline fusion is the most desired method to convert ore to manganates. That is, in the presence of a strong oxidizing agent such as potassium chlorate, pyrolusite is first fused with alkaline to form potassium manganate:

$$MnO_2 + KClO_3 + 6KOH \longrightarrow 3K_2MnO_4 + KCl + 3H_2O$$

Then, potassium manganate is converted to potassium permanganate with disproportionation reaction or oxidation reaction. If dispmportionation reaction is used, acid or CO_2 gas should be added to promote the reaction. For the CO_2 method:

$$3MnO_4^{2-} + 2CO_2 \longrightarrow 2MnO_4^- + MnO_2 + 2CO_3^{2-}$$

After the reaction, MnO_2 is removed by filtration and potassium permanganate crystals are collected through evaporation and concentration. This method is simple and essentially free of contamination. However, the conversion of potassium manganate is only around 2/3 with the rest 1/3 converted to MnO_2.

High purity potassium permanganate is obtained through recrystallization (solubility: 60℃, 22.1g/100g of water; 20℃, 6.34g/100g of water; 0℃, 2.83g/100g of water)

Requirements

(1) Use above method to design the synthesis of potassium permanganate. Identify experimental equipment and demonstrate the synthesis procedures with a flow chart.

(2) After the experimental design being approved by the instructor, carry out the experiment and recrystallize the product.

(3) Calculate the yield.

(4) Complete the experiment report (Principles, Procedures, and Results and Discussion).

Sun Lian

EXERCISE

1. Choice

(1) Which of the following as a chemical reaction?
   a. an iron nail rusts   b. an ice cube melts   c. a limb falls from a tree

(2) Which of the following electron configurations are not possible?
   a. $1s^2 1p^2$ b. $1s^2 2s^2 2p^2$ c. $1s^2 2s^2 2p^6 2d^1$ d. $1s^2 2s^3$

(3) Which of the following would be considered a 'pure' substance?
   a. blood   b. urine   c. saline   d. aspirin

(4) Which of the following numbers is correctly expressed using scientific notation?
   a. 2285   b. 3.667×10^2 c. 34.10×10^{-3} d. 012×10^5

(5) The prefix centi represents what fraction of a basic unit?
   a. 1/10   b. 1/100   c. 1/1000   d. The whole darn thing

(6) How many electrons are in a hydride ion if it has a charge of -1?
   a. 0   b. 1   c. 2   d. 3

(7) How many atoms are contained in a sample of water that weighs 9.008 grams?
   a. 1/2 of Avogadro's number   b. not enough information
   c. avogadros' number   d. 1.5 of Avogadro's number

(8) The maximum number of electrons that can occupy a 4d subshell is:
   a. 4   b. 6   c. 8   d. 10

(9) The ionic compound that forms between aluminum and oxygen has which of the following formula?
   a. AlO_2 b. Al_2O c. Al_2O_3 d. Al_3O e. AlO

(10) Which of the following elements has the highest electronegativity?
   a. B   b. N   c. Si   d. I   e. Cl

(11) What is the proper formula for calcium phosphate?
   a. $CaPO_3$ b. Ca_3PO_3 c. $CaPO_4$ d. Ca_2PO_4 e. $Ca_3(PO_4)_2$

(12) The correct chemical name for SiO_2 is:
   a. silicon dioxide   b. silicon oxide   c. silicon trioxide   d. silicon tetraoxide

(13) How many significant number does 0.010 50 have?
   a. 5   b. 4   c. 6   d. 3

(14) Which are representative metals?
 a. Ca   b. Ag   c. La   d. Cu   e. Zn

(15) Which are metalloids metals?
 a. B   b. Ag   c. La   d. Cu   e. Si

(16) Which of the following groups is correct?
 a. transition metals: Cr, Mn, Fe, Co, Ni, Cu, Zn
 b. metals: Na, Mg, Ag, Au, At, Pb, Si
 c. nonmetals: F, Cl, As, S, Cs, H, Be
 d. main group elements: Mg, Ca, V, Pb, P, S, Y

(17) Which of the following states is incorrect?
 a. we can divide the elements in the periodic table into four categories: ①main group elements, ②transition metals, ③lanthanides, and ④actinides
 b. the Transition Metals are the elements found between the Group IIA Elements and the Group IIB Elements in the periodic table
 c. the transition metals often exhibit only one oxidation state
 d. the transition elements are also known as the d-block elements

(18) Which are not the properties of transition metals?
 a. generally possess metallic luster
 b. softer than Group 1 and Group 2 metals
 c. generally have higher meltingand boiling points and high densities
 d. good conductors of heat and electricity
 e. generally exhibit magnetic properties

(19) The electron configuration of Mn is?
 a. Ar $4s^2 3d^7$ b. Ar $4s^2 3d^3$ c. Ar $3d^5 4s^2$ d. Ar $3d^9$

(20) Which of the following electron configurations is correct?
 a. Sc Ar $3d^1$ b. Cr Ar $3d^5 4s^1$ c. Cu Ar $3d^9 4s^2$ d. Co Ar $3d^8 4s^1$

(21) Which of the following electron configurations is incorrect?
 a. Ti Ar $3d^2 4s^2$ b. V Ar $3d^3 4s^2$ c. Cr Ar $3d^5 s^1$ d. Cu Ar $3d^9 4s^2$

(22) An ionic compound has the formula, $K_2 CrO_4$. What is the oxidation state of chromium in this compound?
 a. +3   b. +5   c. +6   d. +7

(23) Which of the following sequences of atomic radii is true?
 a. Cr > Fe > Co > Ni   b. Ti > Zr > Hf
 c. Mn < Fe < Co < Cu   d. Ni < Pd > Pt

(24) Which of the following elements is not found in nature in the elemental state?

a. Si　　　　　b. C　　　　　c. Ag　　　　　d. S

(25) Which of the following pairs of atoms will form a single covalent bond?
   a. Na and Cl　　b. Mg and Cl　　c. Ne and He　　d. H and F

(26) Which of the following pairs of atoms can form three single bond?
   a. He and He　　b. H and H　　c. N and H　　d. N and N

(27) Which of the following pairs of names and symbols is correct?
   a. silicon tetrafluoride, SiF
   b. nitrogen dioxide, NO
   c. phosphorus trichloride, PCl_3
   d. phosphorus pentachloride, PCl_3

(28) Which of the following molecules is polar?
   a. Oxygen, O_2
   b. Hydrogen iodide, HI
   c. Hydrogen, H_2
   d. Chlorine, Cl_2

(29) Which of the following molecules contains a multiple bond?
   a. methane, CH_4　b. nitrogen, N_2　c. hydrogen, H_2　d. chlorine, Cl_2

(30) The smallest possible unit of a covalent compound is usually considered to be a (an) ?
   a. atom　　　b. cation　　　c. molecule　　　d. polyatomic ion

(31) What type(s) of intermolecular forces, if any, are there between acetic acid molecules?
   a. None
   b. Hydrogen bonding
   c. Dispersion forces
   d. Hydrogen bonding and dispersion forces
   e. All of these

(32) In which molecule is hydrogen bonding likely to be significant?
   a. H_2Se　　b. NH_3　　c. CH_4　　d. All of these　　e. None

(33) Which of the following do you expect to have the highest viscosity?
   a. $CH_3CH_2CH_2CH_2CH_3$　　b. $CH_3CH_2CH_2CH_3$　　c. $CH_3CH_2CH_3$
   d. C_2H_6　　e. None

(34) During which of the following processes does temperature not change?
   a. Melting　　　b. Vaporization　　　c. Sublimation
   d. Condensation　　　e. All of these

(35) In what state of matter do molecules possess the greatest kinetic energy?
   a. solid　　b. liquid　　c. gas　　d. same　　e. none

(36) What is the volume of 2.00 g of carbon dioxide at STP?
   a. 44.8 L　　b. 1.02 L　　c. 1.11 L　　d. 22.4 L　　e. 33.5 L

(37) At what temperature (in °C) will 25.0 g of carbon dioxide (at 1.00 atm) occupy 21.5 L?

　　a. 188 °C　　b. 461 °C　　c. −263 °C　　d. −270 °C　　e. 113 °C

(38) At what temperature will a sample of gas at constant pressure occupy 10.0 L if it occupies 12.4 L at 80.0 °C?

　　a. 285 °C　　b. 11.7 °C　　c. 64.5 °C　　d. 165 °C　　e. 84.5 °C

(39) What would be the new volume of a sample of gas originally at 42.3 L if its pressure were increased from 1.00 atm to 7.35 atm at constant temperature?

　　a. 5.76 L　　b. 1.28 L　　c. 311 L　　d. 0.174 L　　e. 3.28 L

(40) What happens to the mole fraction of oxygen in the air inside a balloon as the air escapes over time?

　　a. It stays the same　　b. It goes down　　c. It goes up

(41) Which of the following is a strong electrolyte?

　　a. H_2O_2　　b. HF　　c. LiF　　d. C_2H_5OH　　e. none

(42) Carbonic acid (H_2CO_3) is a (　　).

　　a. weak electrolyte　　b. nonelectrolyte　　c. strong electrolyte

　　d. all of these　　e. none

(43) Which correctly represents the nuclear equation for beta emission from a ^{40}K nucleus?

　　a. $^{40}_{19}K \rightarrow {}^{40}_{18}Ar + {}^{0}_{1}e$　　　　b. $^{40}_{19}K \rightarrow {}^{40}_{18}Ar + {}^{0}_{-1}e$

　　c. $^{40}_{19}K + {}^{0}_{-1}e \rightarrow {}^{40}_{18}Ar$　　　　d. $^{40}_{19}K \rightarrow {}^{40}_{20}Ca + {}^{0}_{-1}e$

(44) In which direction will the following equilibria be shifted when the pressure is increased by reducing the volume? $2SO_3(g) \rightleftharpoons 2SO_2(g) + O_2(g)$

　　a. to the right　　b. to the left　　c. neither

　　d. all of these　　e. none

(45) In which direction will the following equilibria be shifted when the pressure is reduced by increasing the volume? $CaCO_3(s) \rightleftharpoons CaO(s) + CO_2(g)$

　　a. to the left　　b. to the right　　c. neither

(46) In which direction will the following equilibria be shifted when the pressure is increased by reducing the volume? $2HI(g) \rightleftharpoons H_2(g) + I_2(g)$

　　a. to the right　　b. to the left　　c. neither

(47) For a homogeneous catalysis?

　　a. the reactants must reach the surface

　　b. an enzyme is involved

　　c. one must raise the activation energy

d. the catalyst must be in the same state as the reactants

(48) For a system in equilibrium?
   a. the rate of the forward and reverse reactions are the same
   b. the concentrations of the reactants and products are the same
   c. the solvent must be water
   d. the solution is saturated

(49) Which of the following are present in pure water?
   a. hydronium ions
   b. hydroxide ions
   c. water molecules
   d. all of the above

(50) Which of the following is NOT a properly of an acidic solution ?
   a. changes blue litmus to red
   b. slippery feel
   c. sour taste
   d. has a pH below 7

2. Choice

   a. iced tea
   b. isopropyl alcohol
   c. helium
   d. sugar
   e. potassium

(51) Which is the homogeneous mixture?
(52) Which is the pure substance and compound ?

   a. iced tea
   b. isopropyl alcohol
   c. helium
   d. sugar
   e. blood

(53) Which is the element?
(54) Which is the pure substance?

   a. NaCl
   b. KCl
   c. KOH
   d. NaOH
   e. Na_2O

(55) Which is the potassium chloride?
(56) Which is the sodium hydroxide?

   a. NaCl
   b. KCl
   c. KOH
   d. NaOH
   e. AgCl

(57) Which is the sodium chloride?
(58) Which is the potassium hydroxide?

a. NaCl   b. NaNO₃   c. KNO₃   d. NaOH   e. Na₂O

(59) Which is the sodium nitrate?

(60) Which is the potassium nitrate?

3. Choose right(✓) or wrong(×).

1. A freshly cut surface of sodium quickly becomes dull with a film of white sodium oxide when it is exposed to air, this is a physical change. (   )
2. Milk turning sour is a a physical change. (   )
3. Matter is defined as anything that has mass and occupies space. (   )
4. A chemical reaction is a process of rearranging. Replacing or assign atoms to produce new substances. (   )
5. Orbitals: is a specific region of a sublevel containing a maximum of two electrons. (   )
6. Adding calcium phosphate to pure water will reduce the pH. (   )
7. A mixture of a weak acid and its conjugate base in water results in buffer. (   )
8. Actively growing cells are more likely to be affected by exposure to radioactivity. (   )
9. Buffers act by converting strong bases into weak ones. (   )
10. If energy must be added, the change is endothermic. (   )

4. Fill in the blanks.

1. ____ Elements with little or no tendency to gain or lose electrons often react and achieve noble-gas electronic configurations by sharing electrons.
2. ____ Chemical reactions are conveniently represented by equations in which reading substances, called reactants, and the substances produced, called products, are written in terms of formulas.
3. ____ The properties of elements tend to repeat in a regular (periodic) way when the elements are arranged in order of increasing atomic numbers.
4. ____ The arrangements of electrons in orbitals, subshells, and shells are called electronic configuration.
5. ____ are the outermost electrons in an atom, which have the potential to became involve in the bonding process.
6. ____ atoms are most stability if they have a filled or empty outer layer of electron.
7. ____ how close to the true value.
8. ____ energy released when an atom gain an electron.
9. ____ An extension of the counting by weighing idea leads to the mole concept in

which the number of atoms in a specific sample of an element is determined. The sample size used is a mass in grams equal to the atomic weight of the element. The number of atoms.

10. _____ do result in a change in composition, and can be observed only through chemical reactions.

5. Calculation.

(1) A mixture of 15.0g Al and 40.0g of Fe_2O_3 is prepared. The mixture is heated, and a vigorous reaction occurs according to the balanced equation.

$$Fe_2O_3(s) + 2\ Al(s) \rightarrow Al_2O_3(s) + 2\ Fe(l)$$

How many grams of iron are produced?

(2) Calculate the atomic mass of naturally occurring chlorine if 75.77% of chlorine atom are $^{35}_{17}Cl$ and 24.23% of chlorine atoms are $^{37}_{17}Cl$.

Answers

1. Choice

1. A 2. D 3. D 4. B 5. B   6. C 7. A 8. D 9. C 10. E
11. E 12. A 13. B 14. A 15. E   16. A 17. C 18. B 19. C 20. B
21. D 22. C 23. A 24. A 25. D   26. C 27. C 28. B 29. B 30. C
31. D 32. B 33. A 34. E 35. C   36. B 37. B 38. C 39. A 40. C
41. C 42. A 43. B 44. B 45. B   46. C 47. D 48. A 49. D 50. B
51. A 52. D 53. C 54. B 55. B   56. D 57. A 58. C 59. B 60. C

2. Choose right(√) or wrong(×).

1. F 2. F 3. T 4. T 5. T   6. T 7. T 8. T 9. F 10. T

3. Fill in the blanks.

(1) covalent bonding (2) chemical equations (3) period law (4) electronic configuration (5) valence electron (6) a octet rule (7) accuracy (8) electronic affinity (9) mole (10) chemical property

4. Calculation.

(1) Solution

$$Fe_2O_3(s) + 2\ Al(s) \rightarrow Al_2O_3(s) + 2\ Fe(l)$$
$$40.0g 15.0g$$

Convert each mass of reactant to moles

$$15.0 \text{g Al} \times \frac{1 \text{mol Al}}{27.0 \text{g Al}} = 0.556 \text{mol Al}$$

$$40.0 \text{g Fe}_2\text{O}_3 \times \frac{1 \text{mol}}{159.7 \text{g Fe}_2\text{O}_3} = 0.250 \text{mol Fe}_2\text{O}_3$$

$$0.556 \text{mol Al} \times \frac{1 \text{mol Fe}_2\text{O}_3}{2 \text{mol Al}} = 0.278 \text{mol Fe}_2\text{O}_3 \text{ needed}$$

Use the limiting reactant to calculate the mass of product

$$0.250 \text{mol Fe}_2\text{O}_3 \times \frac{2 \text{mol Fe}}{1 \text{mol Fe}_2\text{O}_3} \times \frac{55.85 \text{g Fe}}{1 \text{mol Fe}} = 27.9 \text{g Fe}$$

Answer: 27.9 grams of iron are produced.

(2) Solution: convert each percentage to a decimal fractio

$$75.77\% \times \frac{1}{100\%} = 0.7577$$

$$24.23\% \times \frac{1}{100\%} = 0.2423$$

contribution to atomic mass by chlorine-35 =
fraction of all Cl atoms that are chlorine-35 × mass of a chlorine-35 atom

$$= 0.7577 \times 35$$

$$= 26.52 \text{amu}$$

contribution to atomic mass by chlorine-37 =
fraction of all Cl atoms that are chlorine-37 × mass of a chlorine-37 atom

$$= 0.2423 \times 37.00$$

$$= 8.965 \text{amu}$$

atomic mass of naturally occurring Cl =
contribution of chlorine-35 + contribution of chloine-37

$$= 26.52 + 8.965$$

$$= 35.49 \text{amu}$$

Answer: the atomic mass of naturally occurring chlorine is 35.49amu.

Ainiwaer

APPENDIX

Table 1 List of atomic weight

at No.	symbol	name	atomic Wt
1	H	Hydrogen	1.00794(7)
2	He	Helium	4.002602(2)
3	Li	Lithium	6.941(2)
4	Be	Beryllium	9.012182(3)
5	B	Boron	10.811(7)
6	C	Carbon	12.0107(8)
7	N	Nitrogen	14.0067(2)
8	O	Oxygen	15.9994(3)
9	F	Fluorine	18.9984032(5)
10	Ne	Neon	20.1797(6)
11	Na	Sodium	22.989770(2)
12	Mg	Magnesium	24.3050(6)
13	Al	Aluminium	26.981538(2)
14	Si	Silicon	28.0855(3)
15	P	Phosphorus	30.973761(2)
16	S	Sulfur	32.065(5)
17	Cl	Chlorine	35.453(2)
18	Ar	Argon	39.948(1)
19	K	Potassium	39.0983(1)
20	Ca	Calcium	40.078(4)
21	Sc	Scandium	44.955910(8)
22	Ti	Titanium	47.867(1)
23	V	Vanadium	50.9415(1)
24	Cr	Chromium	51.9961(6)
25	Mn	Manganese	54.938049(9)
26	Fe	Iron	55.845(2)
27	Co	Cobalt	58.933200(9)
28	Ni	Nickel	58.6934(2)
29	Cu	Copper	63.546(3)
30	Zn	Zinc	65.39(2)
31	Ga	Gallium	69.723(1)

Continutte

at No.	symbol	name	atomic Wt
32	Ge	Germanium	72.64(1)
33	As	Arsenic	74.92160(2)
34	Se	Selenium	78.96(3)
35	Br	Bromine	79.904(1)
36	Kr	Krypton	83.80(1)
37	Rb	Rubidium	85.4678(3)
38	Sr	Strontium	87.62(1)
39	Y	Yttrium	88.90585(2)
40	Zr	Zirconium	91.224(2)
41	Nb	Niobium	92.90638(2)
42	Mo	Molybdenum	95.94(1)
43	Tc	Technetium	[98]
44	Ru	Ruthenium	101.07(2)
45	Rh	Rhodium	102.90550(2)
46	Pd	Palladium	106.42(1)
47	Ag	Silver	107.8682(2)
48	Cd	Cadmium	112.411(8)
49	In	Indium	114.818(3)
50	Sn	Tin	118.710(7)
51	Sb	Antimony	121.760(1)
52	Te	Tellurium	127.60(3)
53	I	Iodine	126.90447(3)
54	Xe	Xenon	131.293(6)
55	Cs	Caesium	132.90545(2)
56	Ba	Barium	137.327(7)
57	La	Lanthanum	138.9055(2)
58	Ce	Cerium	140.116(1)
59	Pr	Praseodymium	140.90765(2)
60	Nd	Neodymium	144.24(3)
61	Pm	Promethium	[145]
62	Sm	Samarium	150.36(3)
63	Eu	Europium	151.964(1)
64	Gd	Gadolinium	157.25(3)
65	Tb	Terbium	158.92534(2)
66	Dy	Dysprosium	162.50(3)

Continute

at No.	symbol	name	atomic Wt
67	Ho	Holmium	164.93032(2)
68	Er	Erbium	167.259(3)
69	Tm	Thulium	168.93421(2)
70	Yb	Ytterbium	173.04(3)
71	Lu	Lutetium	174.967(1)
72	Hf	Hafnium	178.49(2)
73	Ta	Tantalum	180.9479(1)
74	W	Tungsten	183.84(1)
75	Re	Rhenium	186.207(1)
76	Os	Osmium	190.23(3)
77	Ir	Iridium	192.217(3)
78	Pt	Platinum	195.078(2)
79	Au	Gold	196.96655(2)
80	Hg	Mercury	200.59(2)
81	Tl	Thallium	204.3833(2)
82	Pb	Lead	207.2(1)
83	Bi	Bismuth	208.98038(2)
84	Po	Polonium	[209]
85	At	Astatine	[210]
86	Rn	Radon	[222]
87	Fr	Francium	[223]
88	Ra	Radium	[226]
89	Ac	Actinium	[227]
90	Th	Thorium	232.0381(1)
91	Pa	Protactinium	231.03588(2)
92	U	Uranium	238.02891(3)
93	Np	Neptunium	[237]
94	Pu	Plutonium	[244]
95	Am	Americium	[243]
96	Cm	Curium	[247]
97	Bk	Berkelium	[247]
98	Cf	Californium	[251]
99	Es	Einsteinium	[252]
100	Fm	Fermium	[257]
101	Md	Mendelevium	[258]

at No.	symbol	name	atomic Wt
102	No	Nobelium	[259]
103	Lr	Lawrencium	[262]
104	Rf	Rutherfordium	[261]
105	Db	Dubnium	[262]
106	Sg	Seaborgium	[266]
107	Bh	Bohrium	[264]
108	Hs	Hassium	[277]
109	Mt	Meitnerium	[268]
110	Uun	Ununnilium	[281]
111	Uuu	Unununium	[272]
112	Uub	Ununbium	[285]
114	Uuq	Ununquadium	[289]
116	Uuh	Ununhexium	see Note above
118	Uuo	Ununoctium	see Note above

Table 2 The concentration of acid and base used frequently in laboratory

name of solution	density (g/ml, 20℃)	weight fraction %	concentration of amount substance (mol/L)
thick H_2SO_4	1.84	98	18
diluted H_2SO_4	1.18	25	3
	1.06	9	1
thick HNO_3	1.42	69	16
diluted HNO_3	1.20	33	6
	1.07	12	2
thick HCl	1.19	28	12
diluted HCl	1.10	20	6
	1.03	7	2
H_3PO_4	1.7	85	15
thick $HClO_4$	1.7—1.75	70—72	12
diluted $HClO_4$	1.12	19	2
ice HAc	1.05	99	17
diluted HAc	1.02	12	2
thick $NH_3 \cdot H_2O$	0.88	28	15
diluted $NH_3 \cdot H_2O$	0.98	4	2